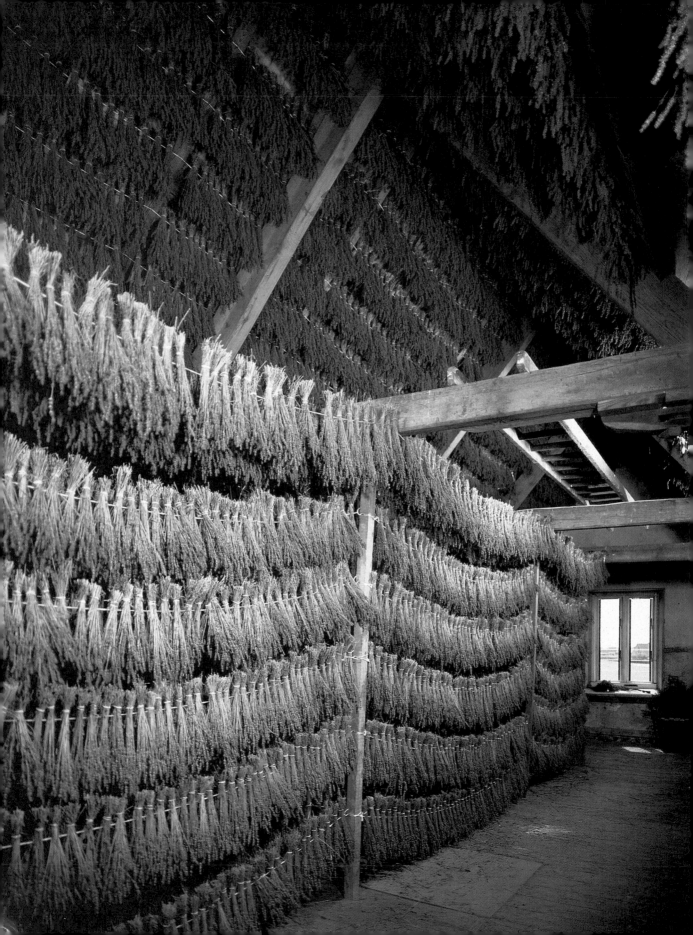

HERBS

— FOR —
COMMON AILMENTS

Anne McIntyre

A GAIA ORIGINAL

A Fireside Book
Published by Simon & Schuster Inc.
New York London Toronto Sydney Tokyo Singapore

A GAIA ORIGINAL

Conceived by	Joss Pearson
Editorial	Joanna Godfrey Wood
	Fiona Trent
Design	Sara Mathews
Photography	Philip Dowell
Illustration	Elaine Franks
Direction	Joss Pearson
	Patrick Nugent

FIRESIDE
Simon & Schuster Building
Rockefeller Center
1230 Avenue of the Americas
New York, New York 10020

FIRESIDE and colophon are registered trademarks
of Simon & Schuster Inc.

Printed in Singapore by Craft Print Pte

Library of Congress Cataloging-in-publication Data
McIntyre, Anne.
        Herbs for common ailments / Anne McIntyre.
            p.   cm.
        "A Gaia original."
        "A Fireside book."
        ISBN 0-671-74632-4
1. Herbs--Therapeutic use. I. Title.
RM666.H33M4 1992
615'.321--dc20   91-8886
                                                CIP

10 9 8 7 6 5 4 3 2 1

CONTENTS

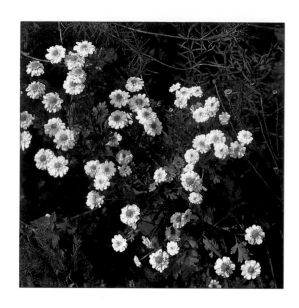

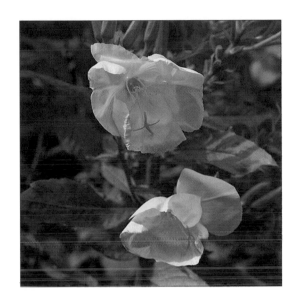

INTRODUCTION

Plants occupy a special place in our lives. We have probably all felt uplifted by the fragrance of a rose, a walk through a poppy field, or the magic of a forest after rain. As global and local ecology become ever-more pressing issues, many of us are increasingly aware of how much we depend on the plant world to sustain us. Plants have always provided us with the raw materials for shelter, transport, clothing, tools, and, traditionally, utensils, and have occupied a central place in mythology and religious ceremonies. They are the source of the food we enjoy, the air we breathe, and for thousands of years have given us herbal medicines with a myriad of therapeutic qualities. As our environment and the plant world become increasingly threatened, the growing realization that we are interdependent with nature is permeating our consciousnesses with greater impact than before.

Despite the move in the nineteenth century toward technological medicine and the use of sophisticated drugs, traditional plant remedies still provide about 85 per cent of the world's medicines. Ancient traditions of medicine, with an energetic perception of the whole person, and systems of healing that utilize plant foods and medicinal herbs, have survived for thousands of years and are as valuable today as they ever were. The recognition of their worth is increasing widely as many people seek a greater understanding of themselves - body, mind, and spirit - and thereby assume more responsibility for their own wellbeing. People are looking for safe, effective, and time-proven alternatives to the modern approach to medicine, with its emphasis on compartmentalizing the body and its symptoms, and symptomatic relief employing largely synthetic drugs. Herbal medicines have soared in popularity and the idea that herbs are synonymous with everything natural and healthy is well established.

Herbal therapy addresses the fundamental concepts of health. Central to herbal philosophy is recognition of the existence of the Vital Force - that energy that flows throughout nature and gives life. Essential to life is the ability to maintain homeostasis - inner balance (of, for example, blood sugar levels, temperature, fluid balance, chemical composition of the blood, and respiration rate) despite constantly varying externals, and to heal ourselves when this balance is disrupted. This innate wisdom, which permeates our every dimension, is the energy of the Vital Force - named in other cultures as Prana and Qi (or Chi).

Disturbance of inner balance causes symptoms to emerge, representing the efforts of the Vital Force to re-establish harmony. To illustrate, a cough is an attempt to clear air passages of irritation or obstruction, and fever enables the body to fight invading pathogens more effectively. To suppress symptoms without due consideration of their significance is to go against the Vital Force. The art of the herbalist is to recognize the efforts of this healing energy and to support and enhance them through the use of plant foods and medicinal herbs.

To provide effective treatment, physical symptoms should be viewed in the context of the individual concerned, their past and their present, their physical body, emotional state and mental attitude, their social, domestic, and working environment, relationships and beliefs, as well as diet, relaxation, and exercise. These all play important parts in the emergence of a person's disease pattern. Diet and nutrition are vital considerations (see pp. 26-9). A natural, wholefood diet is the only one that will provide all that is required generally for energy, health, and the raw materials and building blocks for growth and repair. It is widely accepted that a poor diet can, for example, exacerbate the effects of stress and tension, leading to nervous disorders. The movement back to "real" foods - fresh, plain, and as near their natural state as possible - is gaining momentum. A wholefood diet ensures the best foundation for health and healing.

While it is important to provide symptomatic relief for ailments, it is at all times essential to address the underlying disturbances. With this understanding, the adept, experienced herbalist can formulate a herbal prescription and counsel as to lifestyle, thereby assisting the person's journey of change and self-healing.

The purpose of this book is to provide lay people with sufficient information to prescribe herbs for themselves and others, to redress their common ailments, either beforehand or once the symptoms have emerged and a "diagnosis" established. Herbal medicines, when properly used, are gentle, safe, and effective. They have the benefit of millennia of human experience to verify their effects and efficacy. Humans and plants have always coexisted and our bodies are well adapted to metabolize plant constituents as they occur in nature. Our harmonious relationship with the plant world, enlivened by the same life force, is illustrated by the ability of herbs to provide us with the perfect medicines for so many of our ills.

About this book
The plants featured in this book form a selection of the more easily available herbs that may be used to help cure a wide variety of complaints. Chapter 1 (The Whole Plant) tells you how to prepare and use the herbs, and what doses to take, if applicable. There is also information on the constituents of herbs, diet and nutrition, and a chart where you can see at a glance which herbs can help a particular ailment. In Chapter 2 (The Ailments) the ailments are arranged by body system, with separate sections for children's illnesses and first aid. Italicized words are cross-references.

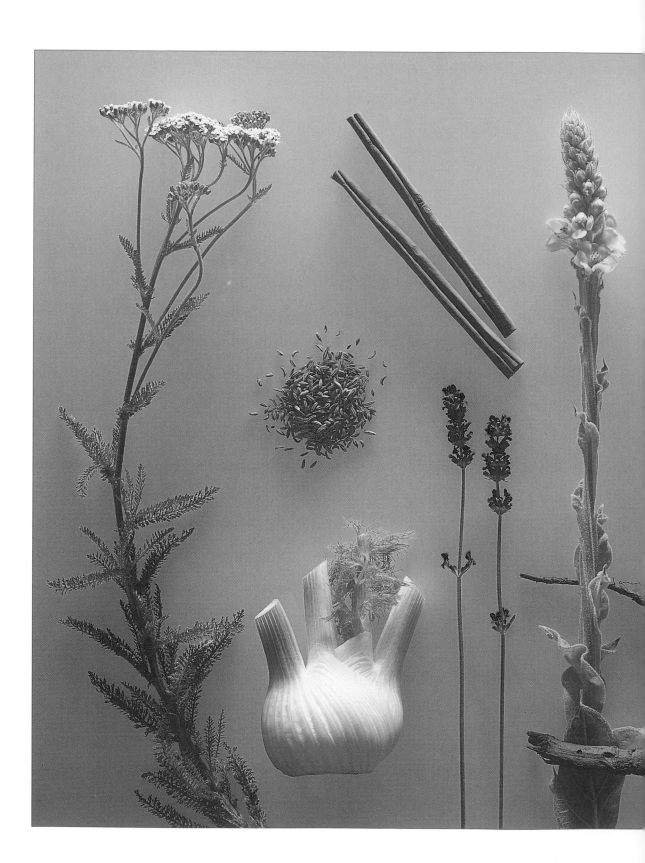

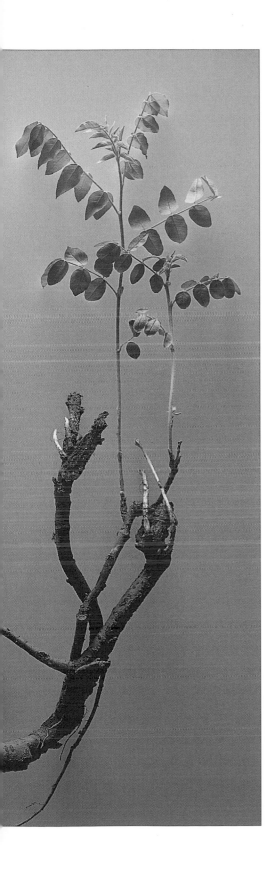

CHAPTER 1

THE WHOLE PLANT

Plants take up substances from the soil and synthesize them into compounds that our bodies can metabolize, use to keep us healthy, and heal us when we fall ill. Vitamins, minerals and trace elements, carbohydrates, proteins, and fats contained in medicinal herbs provide us with the raw materials for health and recovery, while other medicinal agents such as tannins, alkaloids, volatile oils, and bitters work more specifically on certain tissues, organs, and systems to help the healing work of the Vital Force.

There are two different types of medicinal substances found in herbs that have equally important parts to play in the healing process. The primary healing agents are the active ingredients, many of which the pharmaceutical industry continue to use as the basis or model for modern drugs. The other, secondary, compounds in herbs act as catalysts and determine how effective the healing agent will be by making the body more or less receptive to its powers. Most herbs contain several active substances, one of which normally dominates, and it is this which largely determines the choice of remedy. Secondary healing agents should not be overlooked though, since they ensure that the herbs are properly assimilated in the body, and that they buffer any side effects from the active ingredients. For this reason, herbal medicine advocates the use of the plant preparation made from all the substances naturally occurring in the part of the plant used.

THE ACTIVE CONSTITUENTS OF HERBS

Most herbs contain several active substances, however there is usually one dominant constituent, and it is this that largely determines the choice of remedy.

Tannins have a mainly astringent action, binding albumen - a protein found in both the skin and mucous membrane - to form a tight, insoluble layer that protects against irritation and infection. This layer prevents infecting organisms that settle on the skin or mucosae, from gaining access to their source of nutrition, and helps speed healing. Tannins are the main constituents in herbs such as agrimony, witch hazel, eyebright, and raspberry leaves. These herbs may be used as *gargles* for *sore throats*, *mouthwashes*, remedies for *diarrhoea*, *compresses* for *wounds*, and *eyewashes* for *conjunctivitis*.

Volatile oils are found in high concentration in the highly scented herbs. These include rosemary, thyme, sage, basil, dill, fennel, and oregano. The compounds making up these volatile oils vary from one aromatic herb to another, as do their actions. All have antiseptic and antimicrobial properties, supporting the work of the immune system. Many, such as chamomile, have anti-inflammatory and antispasmodic properties which help relieve inflamed and irritated conditions, *tension*, and colicky

pains. Some, such as thyme and hyssop, have expectorant action, helping to expel *mucus/catarrh* from the chest, others are diuretic, while some act as tonics to the stomach, liver, gallbladder, and intestines. There are those that may also act to stimulate the heart and circulation.

Bitters are substances with a bitter taste that affect mainly the digestive tract. They stimulate secretion of digestive juices in the stomach and intestines and the flow of bile in the liver. They are prescribed for poor appetite, weak digestion, *heartburn*, and *indigestion*, *anaemia*, poor liver and gallbladder function, *exhaustion*, and to aid convalescence. Bitters also have other properties. Some are sedative and relaxant; others are anti-inflammatory; and some enhance the function of the immune system, acting as natural antimicrobial and anticancer remedies. Widely used "bitter tonics" include dandelion root, burdock, golden seal, and feverfew.

Mucilage is a sugary, gel-like substance that has the ability to draw water to it, so that when added to water it swells up to form a viscous fluid. Plants containing high proportions of mucilage, such as flax or psyllium seeds, have a mild laxative effect, acting to absorb water into the bowel, bulking out

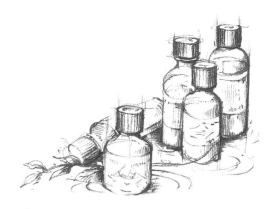

Aromatherapy, the art of using the aromas of volatile oils, has much to offer, not only for physiological imbalances but also for mental and emotional problems. It can be wonderfully helpful in dealing with stress-related disorders.

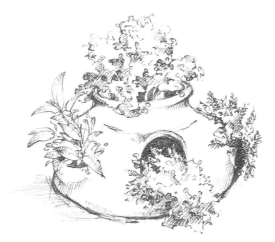

and loosening bowel contents, and thereby helping to propel them along. Remedies such as marshmallow, comfrey, and slippery elm are used for their high mucilage content. The mucilage forms a protective surface on the mucous membranes throughout the body, quickly soothing inflammation and irritation. It also enhances the effects of other healing agents such as tannins, especially in the relief of irritation.

Alkaloids are compounds that contain nitrogen and tend to have quite powerful effects, particularly on the nervous system, often being toxic in large doses. The use of many herbs containing alkaloids is restricted by law to qualified herbalists and doctors, but most of us are aware of the effects of common alkaloids such as caffeine in coffee and nicotine in tobacco. Alkaloids also occur in small, non-toxic amounts in other herbs, where they exist as catalysts to other

healing agents, as in coltsfoot, St John's wort, wood betony, and comfrey.

Flavonoids and bioflavoniods impart a yellow-orange colour to plants such as cowslips and oranges. Most herbs containing flavonoids are diuretic, as in buchu and burdock. Some are antispasmodic and anti-inflammatory, as in licorice, while others are bioflavonoids in vitamin-C-rich plants, such as blackcurrants and citrus fruits.

Saponins are glycosides that form a soap-like lather when mixed with water and act to emulsify oils. Taken orally they are hardly absorbed at all, but they may act to enhance digestion and absorption of other substances such as calcium and silica. Some saponins are diuretic, as in horsetail and asparagus; others are expectorant, as in mullein and cowslips; while some help strengthen blood vessel walls, reducing permeability and fragility. Steroidal saponins are similar in structure to our body's hormones. Herbs containing these are known as adaptogens, the most well known being ginseng. Others include licorice, devil's bit/false unicorn root, squaw vine, black and blue cohosh, and wild yam. **Warning** Saponins can dissolve red blood cells, so should never be used on broken skin or taken by injection.

Bioflavonoids *are found in vitamin-C-rich plants such as blackcurrants and lemons. They act synergistically with ascorbic acid to aid its metabolism and to strengthen and heal blood vessel walls. This is useful in treatment of vascular problems such as* varicose veins, *bleeding, and* high blood pressure.

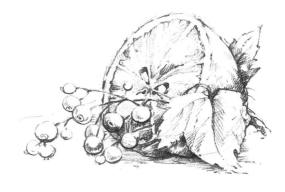

COLLECTING, DRYING, AND STORING

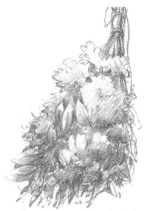

There is no better initiation into the therapeutic world of herbs than a morning walk in spring or summer, when fields and hedgerows are everyone's herbal dispensary, open all hours. The sheer enjoyment of being in their midst and gathering leaves and blossoms, roots and barks for healing, can never be exaggerated.

Always pick herbs away from roadsides or cultivated land that may have been sprayed, and gather them at their most vigorous. Be careful not to overpick the same area, or gather from places where the plant is scarce, and avoid any plant that looks stunted or diseased. Be gentle in your handling of fresh herbs - do not bruise or crush them, or hold them for too long.

For most herbs in spring and summer leaves are at their best just before flowering, and flowers are at their best just as they are bursting into bloom. Bark should be harvested in spring as the sap rises, while roots and rhizomes should be left until fall/autumn. Collect leaves and flowers on a dry, sunny day in the morning, once the dew has dried, as dampness will cause them to deteriorate quickly. Bark, roots, and rhizomes are easier to pull after rain.

As soon as you get home, spread the plants out to dry in a single layer or hang them in small bunches. Choose a warm, airy, well-ventilated place in the shade, such as an attic

or shed. Wash and cut roots and rhizomes only and then dry them. Turn the herbs frequently over the next few days, and when dry, break them up into small pieces. Drying times vary depending on the plant and the part you intend to use. Generally, leaves should be brittle and break easily. Stems and stalks should break and not bend. Flower petals should rustle but not crumble. Bark and roots should be dry enough to snap, or if they are thick, to chip with a small hammer. Dried herbs should look, taste and smell like the fresh plant, but be about one-eighth the weight.

Store the herbs in a dark, dry place, in brown paper bags, cardboard boxes or dark glass jars with cork stoppers - never in plastic because it encourages condensation inside the container. Label the containers carefully. Aerial parts will keep for about a year; roots and bark for two.

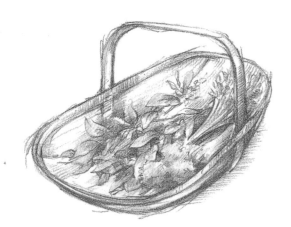

Open baskets *are ideal containers to use when you are collecting herbs - the plants can lie flat without being crushed and bruised. When you get home deal with your harvest straight away and never leave it to deteriorate.*

PREPARATIONS FOR INTERNAL USE

The following three pages give the basic instructions you will need to take internally the herbs recommended in The Ailments section (see pages 30-91).

Tea You can prepare a herbal tea either as an *infusion* or a *decoction* (see below). Choose the infusion method to prepare teas when using the soft aerial parts of plants, such as the flowers and leaves. Use the decoction method to prepare more woody materials such as roots, bark, and seeds.

Infusions are prepared just like Chinese or Indian teas, and are used for soft parts of plants - flowers, stems, and leaves. Make a standard adult dose with 1oz (28g) of dried herb to 1 pint (600ml) of water or a teaspoonful per cup. Double the amount if the herb is fresh. You can vary this according to taste, and halve or quarter it for children. You can also use tea bags from health food stores. Place the herbs in a warmed pot, pour on boiling water and cover to prevent beneficial essential oils from being lost to the atmosphere. Leave to infuse for about 10 minutes and strain. You can either drink it immediately or store it in the refrigerator in an airtight container for up to two days. Herbs with a high mucilage content such as marshmallow or comfrey root need to be made up as cold infusions, otherwise their

therapeutic constituents may be destroyed. Pour cold water over the herb and leave to infuse for 10-12 hours. Generally it is best to take infusions hot by the cupful three times daily in chronic problems and up to every hour or two in acute illness. Children will only be able to take little amounts at a time, so give small amounts often. For urinary tract disorders it is best to drink infusions luke warm to cold. You can combine several herbs together in an infusion, so that aromatic herbs like peppermint, lemon balm, lavender, catnip, and fennel disguise the taste of less palatable herbs. You can also use licorice, aniseed, unsweetened fruit juices, or honey to flavour infusions.

Decoctions The hard, woody parts of plants, such as bark, seeds, roots, rhizomes, and nuts have tough cell walls that require great heat to break them down before they can impart their constituents to water. Break the herbs into small pieces by chopping, crushing, or hammering. Use the same proportions of herb to water as when making *infusions*, and then add a little more water to make up for slight loss, through evaporation, during preparation. Place the herb in a saucepan (not aluminium) and cover with cold water. Bring to the boil, cover, and simmer for 10-15 minutes. Strain, flavour or sweeten as for infusions, and drink hot by

Gruel is a kind of porridge made from mixing powdered herbs, such as slippery elm, with warm milk or water, to make a paste. You can then mix this with oatmeal porridge or honey and take 2-3 times daily.

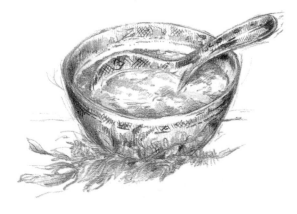

the cupful three times daily for a chronic problem and up to every hour or two for an acute illness.

Syrups You can use syrups to make herbs more palatable, especially for children, or even squeamish adults. Pour 1pt (600ml) of boiling water over 2½lb (1.25kg) of soft brown sugar and stir over gentle heat until all the sugar has dissolved and the solution comes to the boil. If you have herbal *tinctures* you can mix 1 part tincture to 3 parts syrup and this will keep indefinitely. If you prepare an *infusion* or *decoction*, add ¾lb (325g) of sugar to 1pt (600ml) of the liquid and heat until all the sugar dissolves. Cool and store in the refrigerator. Generally give a dessertspoonful to a child 3-4 times daily in chronic problems, and double the dose in acute illness.

Herbal honeys are a delicious and very easy way to give herbal remedies to children. You can chop fresh or dried herbs finely, or powder them and cover with honey. Leave to infuse for a few minutes and then give on a teaspoon. You can also give essential oils in honey - one drop per teaspoon of honey.

Tinctures A mixture of water and alcohol is used to extract the chemical components from the plant and to act as a preservative, making a more concentrated extract of herbs. It has a shelf life of at least two years. The ratio of water to alcohol ranges from 25% alcohol for tannins to 90% alcohol for resins and gums. You can use the herb fresh or dried, either finely chopped or powdered. Place it in a large jar and pour the alcohol and water solution over it. A standard preparation requires one part dried herb to five parts fluid, while fresh herbs can be used at a ratio of 1:2. To make 2.2 pints (1 litre) of chamomile tincture: take 7oz (200g) of dried herb and pour over it 2.2 pints (1 litre) of brandy or vodka. Use an air-tight lid and leave to macerate out of direct sunlight for at least two weeks and shake the jar daily. Then press through a muslin bag (or use a simple wine press), squeezing out as much fluid as you can. Then throw away the herb (it makes excellent compost). Pour the tincture into a dark storage jar and keep it in a cool place.

Alternatively you can use equal parts of glycerol and water to make a syrup-like tincture that is particularly suitable for children. Give 1 teaspoonful three times daily after meals in chronic cases and double the dose for acute illness. Use 10 drops to ½ tsp for children. Dilute with water or fruit juice of your choice.

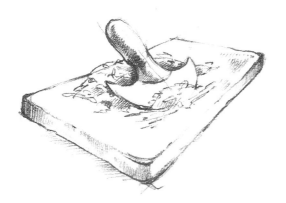

Chopping To make the contents of herbs more accessible, chop them up with a sharp knife when fresh, use a pestle and mortar, or smash them with a hammer if hard.

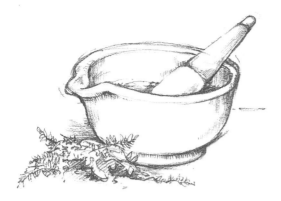

Throat sprays Dilute either 1tsp of tincture or 5 drops of essential oil in half a cup of water or use half a cup of *infusion* or *decoction*. Fill a throat spray, available from most pharmacists/chemists, with this liquid, and spray the back of the throat every 2 hours in acute infections and 3 times daily in chronic problems.

Gargle Dilute 1tsp of herbal *tincture* in half a cup of water, or use half a cup of *infusion* or *decoction*, and gargle every 2 hours in acute infections and 2-3 times daily in chronic problems. Gargle with your head back, holding the liquid in your throat and saying "Aaaah" for a few seconds before spitting the liquid out. Repeat until the liquid is completely finished.

Mouthwash Use 1tsp of herbal tincture diluted in half a cup of water, or half a cup of *infusion* or *decoction*. Rinse it thoroughly around the mouth for a few seconds and then spit it out. Repeat until the liquid is finished. Do this 3 times daily.

Inhalation Using a bowlful of hot *infusion* or *decoction*, or 5-10 drops of essential oil in a bowl of hot water, lean over the steaming liquid, enclosing your head and the bowl with a towel to prevent the steam from escaping. Breathe slowly and deeply to reap the benefit of the remedy for 5-10 minutes. Repeat every 2 hours in acute infections, and twice a day for chronic problems.

Garlic You can take garlic raw, crushed in salads, salad dressings, chopped into honey, or even on toast. For the more squeamish, garlic capsules/perles (as second best) are available from health food stores.

Making tea Infuse the soft aerial parts of the plant, such as the flowers and leaves, for 5-10 minutes, and prepare more woody materials, such as roots and bark, as decoctions by simmering them in boiling water for 5-10 minutes.

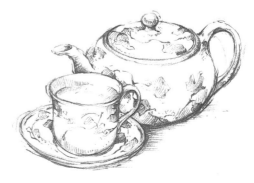

PREPARATIONS FOR EXTERNAL USE

Many ingredients of herbs are easily absorbed through the skin. The preparations for external use described on these two pages are recommended in The Ailments section (see pages 30-91).

Herbal baths Either add a couple of drops of essential oil to the water (use dilute oils for babies and children), hang a muslin bag with fresh or dried aromatic herbs under the hot tap, or add strong herbal *infusions* or *decoctions* to the bath water, and then soak in it for 10-30 minutes. The essential oils are absorbed through the skin pores and inhaled.

Hand and foot baths Use a few drops of essential oil, strong *infusions* or *decoctions*, or a few teaspoons of *tincture* in a bowl of hot water and take a foot bath for 8 minutes in the evening and a hand bath for the same time in the morning. This is an excellent way to give herbs to babies and children.

Ointments, creams, and lotions You can use fresh or dried herbs to make an ointment using this simple recipe: macerate as much herb as you can in 16oz (450ml) of olive oil and 2oz (50g) of beeswax for a few hours over low heat in a bain-marie (water bath for baking gently), during which time chemicals in the herb will be taken up by the oil. Then press the oil out through a muslin bag, and pour it while still warm into ointment jars. You can make creams very easily by mixing either a little *tincture*, *decoction*, *infusion*, or a few drops of essential oil into a base of aqueous cream (from a pharmacist/chemist). Apply ointments and creams 2 to 3 times a day to treat skin problems, *varicose veins* and sore or inflamed joints. Make lotions using herbs in *tinctures*, *infusions*, or *decoctions*, or a few drops of essential oils in water. Apply them externally, 2-3 times daily, for skin problems, *varicose veins*, and for various first aid treatments (see pp.89-91).

Compresses Using either a hot or cold *infusion*, *decoction*, dilute *tincture*, or a few drops of essential oil in water, soak a clean cloth or flannel, then wring it out and apply to the affected part. Repeat applications several times for good effect.

Poultices You can use fresh or dried herbs. Bruise fresh leaves, stems, or roots first, and finely chop or powder dried herbs before adding water to mix into a paste. Then place the paste between two pieces of gauze and bind it to the affected part with a cotton bandage, and keep it warm with a hot water bottle if you can. Leave in place for several hours, and repeat morning and night. Slippery elm will help bring a *boil* to a head

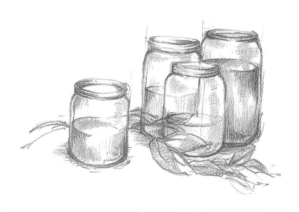

Maceration *Place the herbs in a glass jar with a tight-fitting lid, cover with oil and put it on a sunny window sill. Shake the jar daily. The oil will take up the components of the plants. After two weeks filter off the oil and squeeze the remainder through a muslin bag. Store in a dark bottle in a cool place.*

THE WHOLE PLANT

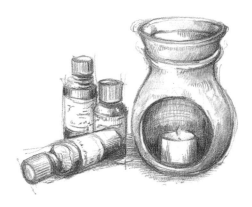

Liniments A liniment, or rubbing oil, is made up of herbal extracts in an oil or alcohol base, or a mixture of *herbal oils* and alcohol *tinctures* of the chosen herbs. Liniments usually contain stimulating essential oils, ginger, or cayenne, to increase local circulation and enhance absorption through the skin.

Herbal oils Although essential oils have to be purchased (see p.93), you can make herbal oils by macerating freshly chopped herbs in pure vegetable oil for about two weeks (see picture, left).

Room spray Dissolve 5-10 drops of essential oil in a little water and put into a plant spray or an atomizer (available from a pharmacy/chemist). Spray the room every few hours if you are ill in bed, or last thing at night before you retire.

Steam treatment/facial steamer Dissolve 5-10 drops of essential oil in a bowl of hot water or in a facial steamer (available from a pharmacy/chemist). Lean over the bowl or steamer, and allow the steam to seep into your skin for 5-10 minutes. Repeat twice a week for skin problems, such as *acne*.

Vaporizers are available in some health food stores and pharmacies/chemists or essential oil suppliers (see p.93). Put a little water into the clay bowl and add 10 drops of your chosen essential oil or blend of a few. Insert a nightlight under the clay bowl – the heat helps the oils to evaporate.

Eyewash/eyebath Using an eyebath from the pharmacist/chemist, half fill it with a luke warm-to-cool *decoction*. Put your head back and hold the eye bath firmly over your open eye. Move your head from side to side for a few seconds so that the remedy rinses the eye thoroughly. Then discard the liquid, wash the eyebath, and use fresh decoction for the other eye. Repeat every 2 hours in acute eye problems and 3 times daily for chronic problems.

Garlic For external use, such as ear drops, crush garlic and then infuse it in vegetable oil for a few hours before straining it.

Sleep pillow Using dried herbs, choose a mixture of relaxing herbs to blend together to your taste. Add a few drops of essential oil if you wish. Fill a small bag or pillow case with the herbs and place it by your head or under your pillow so that you inhale the therapeutic aromas while you sleep.

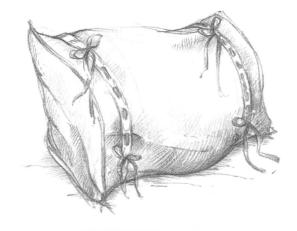

THE MAJOR HERBS AND AILMENTS

To use this chart (pages 20-1), either read from the ailment until you reach a symbol, then up to the herb indicated. Or, read down from the herb to find out which ailments it is likely to help. For treatment instructions, see The Ailments *(pages 30-91).*

Ailment	Burdock	Chamomile	Comfrey	Dandelion	Elderflower	Garlic	Ginger	Ground Ivy	Hawthorn	Lavender	Licorice	Limeflower	Marshmallow	Meadowsweet	Peppermint	Pot Marigold	Rosemary	Sage	Skullcap	St John's Wort	Thyme	Vervain	Wild Oat	Yarrow
IMMUNE SYSTEM																								
FEVERS/INFECTIONS		●		●	●	●	●					●	●	●							●	●		●
ALLERGIES		●	●									●		●										●
CANDIDIASIS		●		●											●		●				●			
ME/POST VIRAL SYNDROME	●	●	●	●							●					●				●	●	●	●	●
HERPES	●	●	●	●		●			●						●				●	●	●	●	●	●
NERVOUS SYSTEM																								
TENSION, ANXIETY, STRESS		●							●	●	●				●			●	●	●		●	●	●
DEPRESSION			●						●									●	●	●		●	●	●
INSOMNIA		●							●	●									●			●		
HEADACHES, MIGRAINE		●				●	●		●		●		●	●			●		●	●		●		●
TIREDNESS, EXHAUSTION	●		●		●	●			●	●						●	●	●			●	●		●
NEURALGIA		●					●		●	●	●		●	●			●		●	●		●		●
RESPIRATORY SYSTEM																								
COLDS, FLU	●	●		●	●	●	●	●		●		●	●	●			●				●			●
MUCUS/CATARRH, SINUS PROBLEMS	●	●	●	●	●	●	●	●		●	●	●	●	●			●				●			●
EARACHE		●			●	●	●			●	●	●	●	●	●					●	●			●
SORE THROAT		●			●	●	●	●		●			●	●	●		●				●		●	●
TONSILLITIS	●	●			●	●	●	●		●	●	●	●	●	●		●				●			●
LARYNGITIS, PHARYNGITIS		●			●	●	●	●		●			●	●			●				●			●
ASTHMA	●	●	●		●	●	●	●			●		●						●		●	●		
HAY FEVER, RHINITIS		●			●	●	●			●	●	●	●								●			●
COUGHS, BRONCHITIS			●		●	●	●	●		●	●	●	●	●							●			●
DIGESTIVE SYSTEM																								
CONSTIPATION	●	●		●		●	●			●			●											
DIARRHOEA		●			●	●	●	●				●	●	●							●			
NAUSEA, VOMITING		●					●		●		●	●	●	●							●			
HEARTBURN, INDIGESTION	●	●	●	●			●		●		●		●	●	●	●	●							●
DIVERTICULITIS		●	●	●		●			●		●		●	●	●									
IRRITABLE BOWEL, SPASTIC COLITIS		●	●								●		●	●	●									
FLATULENCE		●		●		●	●						●	●	●	●					●			●
GASTRITIS, PEPTIC ULCERS		●	●					●	●		●	●	●	●	●				●	●		●		●
GALLSTONES, GALLBLADDER PROBLEMS	●	●		●						●			●	●	●	●						●		●
URINARY SYSTEM																								
CYSTITIS, URETHRITIS	●	●	●		●					●	●	●	●								●		●	●
KIDNEY INFECTION, STONES			●	●		●					●	●	●								●			
WATER RETENTION		●		●							●		●									●		●
CIRCULATORY SYSTEM																								
ANAEMIA	●		●	●			●		●								●		●			●		
POOR CIRCULATION, CHILBLAINS				●	●	●	●		●	●			●	●	●	●				●		●		
CRAMPS		●		●	●	●	●		●	●	●		●	●		●		●			●	●	●	
HARDENING OF THE ARTERIES			●	●	●	●			●		●		●											●
HIGH, LOW BLOOD PRESSURE			●	●	●	●	●		●		●			●		●							●	
VARICOSE VEINS, HAEMORRHOIDS		●			●				●		●	●	●	●	●				●					●
VARICOSE ULCERS		●	●		●			●	●		●		●						●			●		●
BONES, JOINTS, MUSCLES																								
ARTHRITIS, GOUT	●		●	●			●		●	●	●		●	●		●				●				
BACKACHE, SCIATICA		●		●			●		●	●			●			●			●	●		●		

THE WHOLE PLANT

20

Key: symbols indicate which part or parts of the herb is used

- Bulb
- Whole plant
- Flowers
- Roots
- Whole plant / seeds
- Flowering herb
- Leaves
- Petals
- Flowers / berries
- Seeds
- Aerial parts
- Inner bark
- Roots, leaves, and seeds
- Aerial parts of flowering plant
- Leaves and flowering tops

	BURDOCK	CHAMOMILE	COMFREY	DANDELION	ELDERFLOWER	GARLIC	GINGER	GROUND IVY	HAWTHORN	LAVENDER	LICORICE	LIMEFLOWER	MARSHMALLOW	MEADOWSWEET	PEPPERMINT	POT MARIGOLD	ROSEMARY	SAGE	SKULLCAP	ST JOHN'S WORT	THYME	VERVAIN	WILD OAT	YARROW
SKIN AND EYES																								
ECZEMA	●	●	●		●				●	●	●		●			●			●			●	●	●
ABSCESSES, BOILS, CARBUNCLES	●		●			●			●	●	●					●					●			
IMPETIGO	●	●				●			●					●	●				●		●			
WARTS, VERRUCAE	●		●			●				●					●									
RINGWORM, ATHLETE'S FOOT	●			●		●			●					●	●						●			
SCABIES						●			●					●			●	●						
PSORIASIS	●	●	●					●	●	●		●			●			●	●		●	●	●	●
CONJUNCTIVITIS, BLEPHARITIS	●	●		●					●					●										●
EYE STRAIN, TIRED EYES		●			●							●	●	●							●			
STYES	●	●			●				●			●	●	●					●		●			●
ACNE	●	●	●	●	●	●	●		●	●			●	●	●		●			●			●	●
REPRODUCTIVE SYSTEM																								
PMS / PREMENSTRUAL TENSION		●	●						●	●					●		●	●		●	●	●		
PAINFUL PERIODS		●			●				●	●	●		●			●		●	●		●	●		
HEAVY PERIODS										●											●			●
VAGINAL INFECTIONS		●			●				●				●							●				
ENDOMETRIOSIS		●								●					●		●	●			●	●		
MENOPAUSAL PROBLEMS			●					●	●						●	●	●			●	●			
LOW SEX DRIVE, IMPOTENCE		●			●	●			●							●				●	●			
LOW SPERM COUNT			●		●	●			●							●				●	●			
PROSTATE PROBLEMS					●	●			●															
PREGNANCY AND CHILDBIRTH																								
MORNING SICKNESS		●				●			●	●			●	●	●									
CHILDBIRTH		●				●			●															
BREAST-FEEDING PROBLEMS		●	●	●	●				●			●		●						●			●	
CHILDREN'S AILMENTS																								
FEVERS, INFECTIOUS DISEASES	●	●			●	●	●	●	●		●		●	●	●					●	●	●		●
BEDWETTING		●							●		●						●	●				●		
HYPERACTIVITY		●						●									●				●	●		
SLEEPLESSNESS		●							●	●	●				●		●	●		●				
CROUP		●							●	●		●												
WORMS		●		●					●		●	●	●							●				
WHOOPING COUGH		●	●		●	●			●	●	●	●	●				●			●				
DIARRHOEA		●	●		●	●	●		●		●	●	●	●		●	●			●			●	●
COLIC		●	●			●	●		●		●	●	●	●		●				●				●
FIRST AID																								
BRUISES			●													●								●
MINOR BURNS, SCALDS		●	●		●				●							●				●				
MINOR CUTS, WOUNDS		●	●				●		●					●		●				●				●
SPLINTERS	●	●	●			●			●			●				●				●				
TOOTHACHE		●							●		●								●	●		●	●	
TRAVEL SICKNESS		●					●		●				●	●		●			●					●
SPRAINS, STRAINS		●	●				●		●					●	●	●				●				
INSECT BITES, STINGS		●	●		●	●			●					●	●	●								●
FAINTING, SHOCK		●			●		●		●							●			●					
NOSE BLEEDS					●									●						●				●

THE SUBSIDIARY HERBS AND AILMENTS

To use this chart (pages 22-5), either read from the ailment until you reach a symbol, then up to the herb indicated. Or, read down from the herb to find out which ailments it is likely to help. For treatment instructions, see The Ailments *(pages 30-91).*

Ailment	Agrimony	Aloe Vera	Arnica	Balmony	Black Cohosh	Black Haw	Blue Cohosh	Boneset	Borage	Brown Beth	Buchu	Catnip	Celandine	Celery Seed	Chickweed	Cinnamon	Cleavers	Coltsfoot	Corn Silk	Couch Grass	Cramp Bark	Devil's Bit	Devil's Claw	Echinacea	Elecampane
IMMUNE SYSTEM																									
Fevers/infections								•								>								•	
Allergies									•															•	
Candidiasis																>								•	
ME/post viral syndrome																•								•	
Herpes									•							•							•	•	
NERVOUS SYSTEM																									
Tension, anxiety, stress									•			•				>					•				
Depression									•							>									
Insomnia												•									•				
Headaches, migraine																>					•	•			
Tiredness, exhaustion																								•	
Neuralgia				•												>					•			•	
RESPIRATORY SYSTEM																									
Colds, flu						•		•				•				>								•	
Mucus/catarrh, sinus problems												•				>	•	○						•	•
Earache												•					•							•	
Sore throat																	•	○						•	
Tonsillitis							•					•					•	○						•	•
Laryngitis, pharyngitis				•								•					•	○						•	•
Asthma									•								•	○						•	•
Hay fever, rhinitis									•			•				>								•	
Coughs, bronchitis									•			•				>		○		•				•	•
DIGESTIVE SYSTEM																									
Constipation				•												>				•					
Diarrhoea	•															>									
Nausea, vomiting	•															>								•	
Heartburn, indigestion																									
Diverticulitis	•																							•	
Irritable bowel, spastic colitis	•																								
Flatulence																>									
Gastritis, peptic ulcers																									
Gallstones, gallbladder problems	•												•												
URINARY SYSTEM																									
Cystitis, urethritis									•		•			•			•		•	•				•	
Kidney infection, stones									•		•			•			•		•	•				•	
Water retention									•		•			•			•		•	•		•			
CIRCULATORY SYSTEM																									
Anaemia									•						•										
Poor circulation, chilblains		•														>									
Cramps																>					•				
Hardening of the arteries									•																
High, low blood pressure														•		>	•			•					
Varicose veins, haemorrhoids		•	•																						
Varicose ulcers																	•			•				•	
BONES, JOINTS, MUSCLES																									
Arthritis, gout					•		•		•					•		>							•	•	
Backache, sciatica																				•	•			•	

Key: symbols indicate which part or parts of the herb is used

- Flowering herb
- Leaves and bark
- Twigs and leaves
- Leaves
- Bark
- Seeds
- Leaves and flowers
- Roots and rhizomes
- Tuber and rhizome
- Leaves, flowers and berries
- Root bark, stem and trunk
- Aerial parts of flowering plant
- Stem bark
- Aerial parts
- Leaves, flowers and seeds

	AGRIMONY	ALOE VERA	ARNICA	BALMONY	BLACK COHOSH	BLACK HAW	BLUE COHOSH	BONESET	BORAGE	BROWN BETH	BUCHU	CATNIP	CELANDINE	CELERY SEED	CHICKWEED	CINNAMON	CLEAVERS	COLTSFOOT	CORN SILK	COUCH GRASS	CRAMP BARK	DEVIL'S BIT	DEVIL'S CLAW	ECHINACEA	ELECAMPANE
SKIN AND EYES																									
Eczema		●							●						●		●	●						●	
Abscesses, boils, carbuncles	●													●			●							●	
Impetigo														●	●		●			●				●	
Warts, verrucae													●											●	
Ringworm, athlete's foot													●				●							●	
Scabies																	●							●	
Psoriasis									●					●	●		●							●	
Conjunctivitis, blepharitis									●								●								
Eye strain, tired eyes																									
Styes																	●							●	
Acne		●															●						●	●	
REPRODUCTIVE SYSTEM																									
PMS/ premenstrual tension														●			●			●	●		●		
Painful periods					●	●	●														●		●		
Heavy periods	●						●			●													●		
Vaginal infections																	●							●	
Endometriosis					●	●	●		●	●							●				●		●	●	
Menopausal problems					●		●														●		●		
Low sex drive, impotence																●									
Low sperm count														●											
Prostate problems														●						●	●		●	●	
PREGNANCY AND CHILDBIRTH																									
Morning sickness																●					●	●			
Childbirth					●	●	●														●	●			
Breast-feeding problems									●						●		●							●	
CHILDREN'S AILMENTS																									
Fevers, infectious diseases									●			●					●							●	
Bedwetting																			●	●					
Hyperactivity									●			●									●				
Sleeplessness												●													
Croup									●			●						●							●
Worms			●																						
Whooping cough									●			●						●							●
Diarrhoea	●											●				●								●	
Colic												●				●									
FIRST AID																									
Bruises			●																						
Minor burns, scalds		●													●					●				●	
Minor cuts, wounds			●																	●				●	
Splinters																									
Toothache																								●	
Travel sickness																●									
Sprains, strains			●																						
Insect bites, stings			●													●									
Fainting, shock			●																						
Nose bleeds																									

	Eyebright	Fennel	Feverfew	Ginseng	Golden Seal	Hops	Hyssop	Lemon Balm	Motherwort	Mullein	Nettle	Passionflower	Plantain	Raspberry	Red Clover	Slippery Elm	Squaw Vine	Thuja	Valerian	Vitex	Wild Yam	Witch Hazel	Wood Betony	Yellow Dock
IMMUNE SYSTEM																								
Fevers/infections					●		●	●																
Allergies					●			●			●				●	●								
Candidiasis					●		●																	
ME/post viral syndrome				●														●						●
Herpes				●		●		●	●		●	●			●				●				●	
NERVOUS SYSTEM																								
Tension, anxiety, stress				●		●		●	●			●			●		●		●	●			●	
Depression				●				●															●	
Insomnia				●		●		●				●							●					
Headaches, migraine			●			●		●				●							●	●			●	
Tiredness, exhaustion				●	●						●		●		●									
Neuralgia				●	●							●							●		●		●	
RESPIRATORY SYSTEM																								
Colds, flu					●		●																	
Mucus/catarrh, sinus problems	●				●		●	●		●			●			●								
Earache					●	●	●	●		●														
Sore throat					●					●			●	●										
Tonsillitis					●		●	●		●			●	●	●									
Laryngitis, pharyngitis		●			●		●			●			●											
Asthma					●		●			●		●			●	●			●					
Hay fever, rhinitis	●		●		●		●	●				●												
Coughs, bronchitis		●					●			●			●		●									
DIGESTIVE SYSTEM																								
Constipation					●																●			●
Diarrhoea		●						●					●	●		●					●			
Nausea, vomiting		●		●	●			●			●					●					●			
Heartburn, indigestion		●		●	●			●								●								
Diverticulitis		●		●				●								●					●			
Irritable bowel, spastic colitis		●		●	●			●								●					●			
Flatulence		●						●													●			
Gastritis, peptic ulcers				●	●			●								●					●			
Gallstones, gallbladder problems		●						●											●		●			
URINARY SYSTEM													●											
Cystitis, urethritis													●											
Kidney infection, stones																								
Water retention													●									●		
CIRCULATORY SYSTEM																								
Anaemia					●						●		●			●								●
Poor circulation, chilblains																								
Cramps					●						●	●							●					
Hardening of the arteries																								
High, low blood pressure								●	●		●	●							●					
Varicose veins, haemorrhoids					●																	●		
Varicose ulcers					●											●								
BONES, JOINTS, MUSCLES																								
Arthritis, gout			●								●										●			●
Backache, sciatica				●				●				●							●					●

Key: symbols indicate which part or parts of the herb is used

- Flowering herb
- Leaves
- Leaves and flowers
- Leaves, flowers and berries
- Stem bark
- Leaves and bark
- Bark
- Roots and rhizomes
- Root bark, stem and trunk
- Aerial parts
- Twigs and leaves
- Seeds
- Tuber and rhizome
- Aerial parts of flowering plant
- Leaves, flowers and seeds

	Eyebright	Fennel	Feverfew	Ginseng	Golden Seal	Hops	Hyssop	Lemon Balm	Motherwort	Mullein	Nettle	Passionflower	Plantain	Raspberry	Red Clover	Slippery Elm	Squaw Vine	Thuja	Valerian	Vitex	Wild Yam	Witch Hazel	Wood Betony	Yellow Dock
SKIN AND EYES																								
Eczema								✓			✓				✓				✓					✓
Abscesses, boils, carbuncles											✓				✓	✓								✓
Impetigo					✓						✓		✓		✓									✓
Warts, verrucae											✓				✓			✓						✓
Ringworm, athlete's foot					✓						✓				✓			✓						✓
Scabies					✓	✓																		
Psoriasis								✓		✓	✓				✓				✓		✓			✓
Conjunctivitis, blepharitis	✓				✓			✓					✓	✓					✓					
Eye strain, tired eyes	✓												✓						✓				✓	
Styes	✓				✓			✓			✓				✓							✓		
Acne								✓			✓		✓		✓						✓	✓		✓
REPRODUCTIVE SYSTEM																								
PMS / premenstrual tension								✓		✓		✓			✓		✓		✓	✓	✓			
Painful periods								✓		✓					✓		✓			✓	✓			
Heavy periods					✓						✓				✓		✓							
Vaginal infections					✓												✓							
Endometriosis					✓			✓		✓		✓			✓		✓		✓	✓	✓	✓		
Menopausal problems				✓				✓		✓		✓								✓				
Low sex drive, impotence			✓								✓				✓					✓				
Low sperm count			✓								✓													
Prostate problems																								
PREGNANCY AND CHILDBIRTH																								
Morning sickness		✓			✓			✓							✓	✓					✓			
Childbirth			✓							✓					✓		✓				✓			
Breast-feeding problems		✓									✓				✓	✓					✓	✓	✓	
CHILDREN'S AILMENTS																								
Fevers, infectious diseases					✓		✓	✓																
Bedwetting								✓																
Hyperactivity						✓		✓			✓	✓			✓				✓					
Sleeplessness						✓		✓				✓							✓					
Croup							✓	✓		✓					✓				✓					
Worms		✓																						
Whooping cough										✓		✓			✓									
Diarrhoea		✓						✓					✓			✓					✓			
Colic		✓			✓			✓				✓				✓					✓			
FIRST AID																								
Bruises																						✓		
Minor burns, scalds					✓																	✓		
Minor cuts, wounds					✓								✓									✓		
Splinters																✓								
Toothache							✓					✓							✓					
Travel sickness		✓						✓																
Sprains, strains																						✓		
Insect bites, stings													✓									✓		
Fainting, shock							✓	✓																
Nose bleeds																						✓		

THE SUBSIDIARY HERBS AND AILMENTS

25

DIET AND NUTRITION

Foods are medicines, preventative and therapeutic, and their energy and vitality can profoundly affect the balance of our energies and our life force. The food we take needs to reflect our requirements, which vary according to age, lifestyle, level of activity, stress, the weather, our state of health, and also factors such as pregnancy or lactation.

Sources	Functions	Supplements
Proteins, first class: meat, poultry, fish, eggs, milk, soya products **Second class:** nuts and seeds, beans and pulses, grains. 2 out of the 3 groups must be combined	Form the basic building blocks of all body tissues, including hormones and antibodies	Ample supply is necessary, particularly in childhood, adolescence, pregnancy, and lactation
Fats (*essential fatty acids*) Seeds, nuts, pulses, beans, unrefined vegetable oils, oily fish, fish liver oils	Vital to normal development of nervous and immune systems. Form the major structural part of the cell wall in every cell in the body. Necessary for absorption of trace elements and fat-soluble vitamins A, E, D, and K	Useful in disturbances of ovulation and menstruation, raised blood cholesterol levels, atherosclerosis, hypertension, and multiple sclerosis. Cod liver oil – 1 tablespoon daily, and evening primrose oil – 500mg daily
Saturated fats Dairy produce, meats, processed fats, refined oils	Provide concentrated energy, insulation, and protection. But excessive amounts predispose to cardiovascular problems and obesity	
Carbohydrates Wholegrains, fruits, vegetables, nuts, seeds, pulses, beans	Complex carbohydrates reduce the risk of cardiovascular disease	
Vitamin A Fish oils, milk produce, (organic) liver, egg yolk, carrots (carotene is found in green, yellow, and orange vegetables and in orange and yellow fruits)	Builds resistance to infections, promotes growth, healthy hair, teeth, skin, gums, tissue repair. Needed for healthy eyes, bone formation, digestion, red/white blood cell production.	To prevent infections and help resolve acute respiratory infections, boils and infections, such as impetigo. Good for weak eyes and hyperthyroidism. Take in cod liver oil – 1 tablespoonful daily
Vitamin B1 (*thiamine*) Wholegrains, oatmeal, (organic) liver, legumes, yeast, milk, nuts, lentils, seeds, eggs	Essential for metabolism of carbohydrates to glucose or fat, and for energy production	Helps recovery from infections or emotional problems. Can relieve fatigue, neuralgia, depression, headaches, irritability. 10-50mg daily in B-complex.

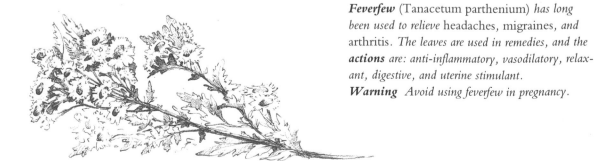

Feverfew (Tanacetum parthenium) *has long been used to relieve* headaches, migraines, *and* arthritis. *The leaves are used in remedies, and the* **actions** *are: anti-inflammatory, vasodilatory, relaxant, digestive, and uterine stimulant.*
Warning *Avoid using feverfew in pregnancy.*

Sources	Functions	Supplements
Vitamin B2 (*riboflavin*) Milk, cheese, butter, yogurt, cereals, meat, wheatgerm, green leafy vegetables, beans, peas, eggs	Involved with formation of liver enzymes and use of oxygen in energy metabolism of carbohydrates, fats, and proteins stored in the liver	Increase in times of growth and with a high-protein diet. Useful for sore tongue and lips, sensitivity to light, and skin problems. 10–20mg daily in B-complex
Vitamin B3 (*nicotinic acid/niacin*) Wholegrains, milk produce, meat, fish, green vegetables, nuts, eggs	Involved with formation of enzymes necessary for carbohydrate metabolism. Affects cholesterol metabolism and helps reduce blood fats	Deficiency is linked to high alcohol consumption and low protein intake. For skin problems, diarrhoea, mouth ulcers, sore tongue, poor appetite, tension, headaches, poor memory. 50mg daily in B-complex/yeast
Vitamin B5 (*pantothenic acid*) Cows' milk, breast milk, eggs, cereals, meat, green vegetables, mushrooms	Involved with metabolism of carbohydrates, fats, and amino acids. The adrenal glands depend on it to function normally and to produce adequate adrenal hormones. Helps the immune system	Increase during pregnancy, lactation, illness, injury, healing and emotional stress. Useful for insomnia, depression cramps, digestive disturbance, nausea and vomiting, numbness and tingling, arthritis and gout. 5–10mg daily in B-complex
Vitamin B6 (*pyridoxine*) Fish, meat, egg yolk, wholegrains, nuts and seeds, green vegetables, bananas, avocados, molasses, mushrooms	Involved in metabolism of proteins and amino acids, sugars, and fatty acids, and some minerals. Aids manufacture of red blood cells, antibodies, hormones, and enzymes	For prevention of cardiovascular disease and skin disease, inflammatory conditions and immune problems. Needs are increased by high protein intake. 5–10mg daily
Vitamin B12 (*cyanocobalamin*) Meat, liver, kidney, fish, eggs, milk produce, beansprouts	For normal development of red blood cells, for metabolism, and healthy nervous system	For symptoms linked to the nervous system, menstrual irregularities, back pain, tiredness, bowel problems, skin disorders. 3–4mg of B-complex daily
Folic acid Green vegetables, eggs, wholegrains, meat, nuts, milk	For red blood cell formation in bone marrow. For metabolism of sugar and amino acids, and manufacture of antibodies. Crucial to normal function of the nervous system. For production of RNA and DNA	Increase in pregnancy, lactation, times of growth and stress, with the Pill, alcohol, and some drugs. 400–800mg daily for anaemia, fatigue, dizziness, depression, susceptibility to infection, sore tongue and mouth

Couch grass (Agropyron repens) *is a curse to gardeners, but a blessing to herbalists. The rhizome is the part of the plant used, and the* **actions** *are: demulcent, soothing and antiseptic, diuretic, calming for pain and spasm in the urinary tract, and antimicrobial.*

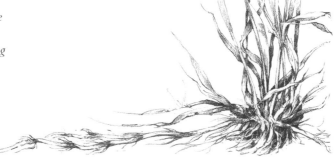

Sources	Functions	Supplements
Vitamin C Fresh fruit and vegetables, potatoes, leafy herbs, and berries	Vital for healthy skin, bones, muscles. Also for healing and protection from the effects of viruses, toxins, drugs, allergies, and foreign bodies.	For poor resistance, fatigue, tender muscles/joints. Increase during stress, infection, surgery, drug therapy, smoking/drinking. 500-1000mg daily
Vitamin D (synthesized in the skin from sunlight) Milk produce, eggs, fatty fish, fish oil	Vital for normal calcium formation and growth and health of bones and teeth. Increases calcium/phosphate absorption	For hot flushes, night sweats, bone fragility, tooth decay, cramps, depression. Cod liver oil – 1 des. spoon daily
Vitamin E Nuts and seeds, eggs, milk produce, wholegrains, wheatgerm, unrefined oils, leafy vegetables, avocados, seaweeds, soya beans, breast milk	For metabolism of essential fatty acids, absorption of iron for red blood cell manufacture. Antioxidant, protects circulatory system, cells, slows ageing. Increases fertility, protects against foetal abnormalities, miscarriage	For wound healing, vascular problems, for menopausal flushes. Avoid if on anticoagulants or with high blood pressure, diabetes, hyper-thyroidism, pregnancy toxaemia. Separate iron from vit. E supplements by 8 hours
Vitamin K Green vegetables, milk products, molasses, apricots, wholegrains, cod liver/sunflower oil, garlic	For production of blood-clotting factors	
Sodium Most vegetables, salt	Vital for fluid balance, blood pressure, normal nerve and muscle function	Increase for vomiting, dizziness, cramps caused by excessive sweating.
Calcium Milk produce, green vegetables, eggs, nuts, seeds, dried fruit, soya beans, bony fish, cereals	For healthy bones and teeth, normal function of heart muscle, blood clotting mechanisms, conduction of nerve impulses, and muscle function	For muscle pain, cramps, PMS/PMT, period/growing pains, osteoporosis, back pains, insomnia, tension, indigestion, constipation. 4-500mg daily
Iron Egg yolk, liver, meat, molasses, soya beans, wholegrains, green vegetables, fish, dried fruits, and wine	Used in production of haemoglobin, vital for oxygen transport in blood. For energy production, cellular respiration, growth/protein metabolism	For anaemia, weakness, headaches, palpitations, depression, poor memory. Increase in pregnancy/lactation, growth/repair periods. 10-20mg daily
Magnesium Green vegetables, nuts, seeds, wholegrains, pulses, potatoes, milk produce, eggs, seafoods, "hard" water	For energy production, protein metabolism, manufacture of enzymes, nerve/muscle function, bone/teeth formation	For convulsions, insomnia, leg/foot cramps, depression, hyperactivity, muscle weakness. Increase for diarrhoea, excessive urination, alcoholism, pregnancy. 300-400mg daily

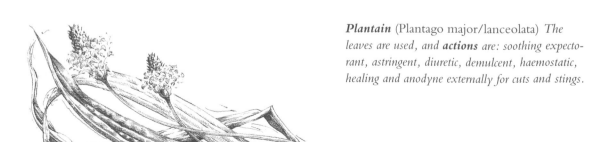

Plantain (Plantago major/lanceolata) *The leaves are used, and* **actions** *are: soothing expectorant, astringent, diuretic, demulcent, haemostatic, healing and anodyne externally for cuts and stings.*

Sources	Functions	Supplements
Phosphorus Wholegrains, seeds, nuts, meat, fish, eggs	For healthy bone formation, heart/kidney function, nerve production and vitamin metabolism	
Potassium Fresh fruit and vegetables, wholegrains, nuts, soya beans, milk, seafood	For nerve conduction and muscle function, to regulate acid/alkali balance of blood/water balance.	Increase with diuretics. For muscle weakness/cramps, low blood sugar, constipation. Use salt substitutes.
Copper Green vegetables, liver, seafood, wholegrains	For formation of myelin sheath, iron, enzyme production, development of brain, bones and with B6, of connective tissue. Acts as an antioxidant. Essential for use of vitamin C	Increase in pregnancy, kidney disease, hypertension, diets high in milk produce, saturated fats and sugar. For high cholesterol levels and other cardiovascular problems. 2-5mg daily
Zinc Oysters, herrings, yeast, liver, eggs, beef, peas, seeds, fruit and vegetables, nuts, poultry, shellfish	For protein metabolism, helps prevent free-radical damage of the eyes, prostate, seminal fluid, and sperm. For normal immune function and hormone production, and healthy bones and joints. Required for release of vitamin A from liver stores	For infection, allergies, auto-immune disease, skin problems, joint pain, menstrual problems, taste/smell loss, coeliac disease, stomach ulcers, ulcerative colitis, hyperactivity. Increase for infections, diabetes, liver disease, smoking/alcohol, drugs. 15mg daily
Cobalt Fruit and vegetables, meat, wholegrains, nuts	Helps copper absorption, magnesium/sugar metabolism	
Manganese Green vegetables, seeds, wholegrains, pulses, eggs, fruits, tea	For energy metabolism, healthy bones, thyroid function, nervous/reproductive systems	For poor growth, anaemia, nervous disorders, learning difficulties. 10-20mg daily of manganese chloride
Iodine Vegetables grown on iodine-rich soils, fruits, seafood, garlic, parsley, iodized salt	Vital to production of thyroid hormones, regulates metabolism, physical/mental development	For low thyroid production, low libido, low blood pressure, weight gain, high cholesterol. Kelp, iodized salt
Chromium Fruit/vegetables, meat, molasses, wholegrains, wheatgerm	Vital for fat and carbohydrate metabolism and production of energy	For diabetes, high blood pressure, arteriosclerosis
Selenium Garlic, wholegrains, eggs, meat	For liver function, connective tissue and formation of sex hormones	For infertility, allergies, joint/muscle problems. Take on a doctor's advice

Cleavers (Galium aparine) *is a reliable diuretic. The aerial parts of the plant are used, and the* **actions** *are: diuretic, antilithic, urinary antiseptic, alterative (working particularly on the lymphatic system), anti-inflammatory, tonic, astringent, antineoplastic, febrifuge, and hypotensive.*

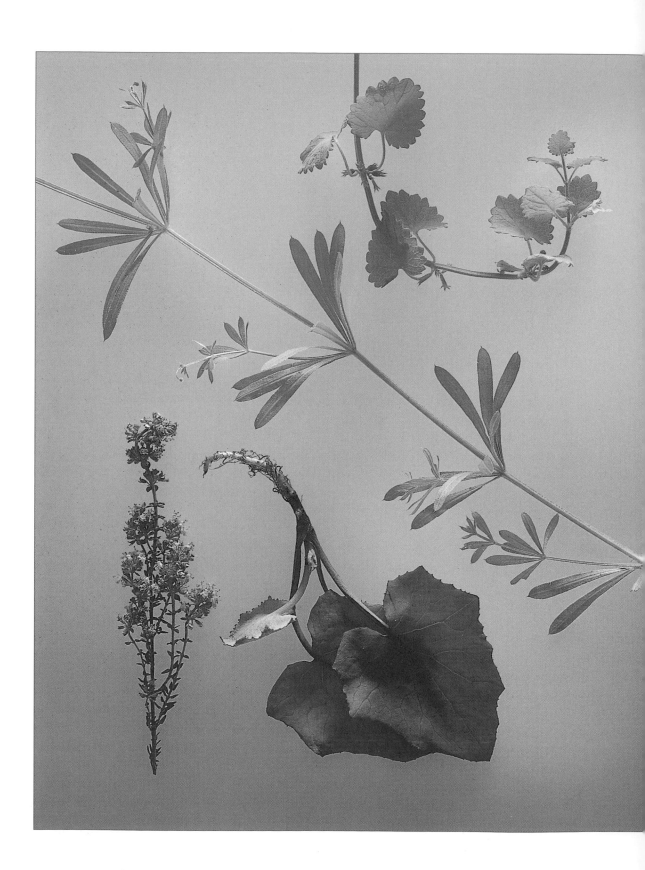

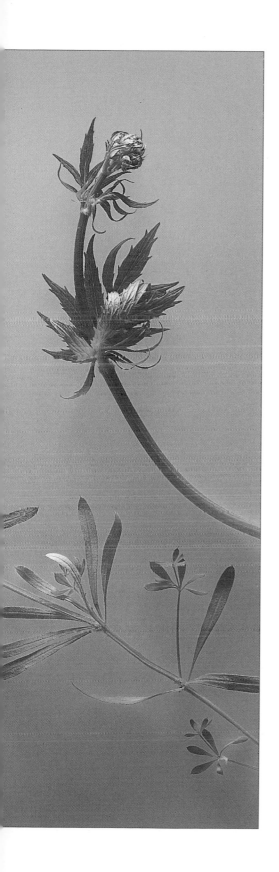

CHAPTER 2

THE AILMENTS

We all possess an inherent ability to restore balance, to repair and heal ourselves when we are ill, thanks to the energy of the Vital Force, and all symptoms of "disease" are a manifestation of this. Herbal remedies can be used to great effect to enhance our own healing process – to help the body to help itself – so that during infections, for example, herbs such as echinacea and garlic can be taken to enhance the function of the immune system, which can then resolve the infection with greater ease. We need to work with the body, not against it.

When treating common ailments at home, it is important to establish the underlying causes of the symptoms, to understand what the Vital Force is attempting to rebalance, and use the herbs accordingly. Otherwise you will simply be providing symptomatic treatment, which will at best temporarily allay the symptoms and suppress healing, only to find that the symptoms recur later or gradually get worse.

It is important to look at each person and their symptoms individually, so that the person is treated, not the disease. People's lives, personalities and psychological make-up, diet, and lifestyle are all different, and all these factors need to be considered when choosing the right herbs for any given ailment. Used in the right way, in conjunction with any necessary changes in diet and lifestyle, herbal remedies can provide good preventative measures, and safe and effective treatment for a wide variety of ailments.

THE IMMUNE SYSTEM

The key to a robust immune system lies in a healthy lifestyle, with nutritious food (see pp.26-9) and a minimum of stress and pollution. Adequate amounts of protein, essential fatty acids, vitamins A, B, C, E, and minerals: copper, iron, magnesium, selenium, and zinc are vital to normal production of white blood cells and antibodies. Immunity can be boosted by increasing intake of these and by immune-enhancing herbs such as garlic, echinacea, licorice, and ginseng.

FEVERS AND INFECTIONS

Fever is a symptom of the body's fight against infection, helping to resolve it, and should not be suppressed (except for fevers in children, see p.84). At the first sign, fast to boost the immune system and drink plenty to assist elimination. Take raw *garlic* in honey, perles, or juice every 2-3 hours, mixed with licorice. Take frequent hot herbal *teas* of limeflower, boneset, chamomile, elderflower, yarrow, and peppermint, singly or in combinations, to hasten elimination of heat and toxins. Hot drinks of lemon and honey, blackcurrant, or beetroot juice increase resistance and provide extra vitamin C. Use essential oils of lavender, chamomile, and eucalyptus in *herbal baths*, *hand and foot baths*, and *inhalations*.

ALLERGIES

When the immune system reacts against non-infectious substances, there is an allergic response as the body attempts to eliminate the allergens. Treatment involves improving nutrition (see pp.26-9), temporarily avoiding the allergen, and balancing the digestive and immune systems. You may need to take, either as *teas* or *tinctures*, a combination of echinacea, red clover, and borage with licorice 3 times daily over several months. You can add marshmallow or slippery elm to soothe the digestive tract, and dandelion root to support the liver and the digestive tract. Chamomile and yarrow tea is a natural antihistamine to take frequently with acute allergies. Nettles in teas or soup help calm the allergic response.

CANDIDIASIS

Candida albicans (or thrush) flourishes when the immune system is weakened by infection, diabetes, long-term or repeated antibiotics, oral contraceptives, steroids, and nutritional deficiencies (see pp.26-9), particularly of iron and zinc. Pregnant women are prone to vaginal thrush and may pass it on

Quantities: See pages 15-19

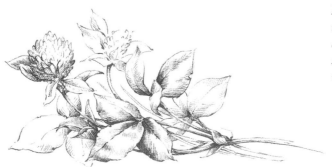

Red clover (Trifolium pratense) *The flowers are used, and the **actions** are: relaxant, expectorant, alterative (particularly good for use in childhood skin conditions), anti-spasmodic, diuretic, and convalescent.*

to the baby. It can also affect the digestive tract, causing general illness, and food and yeast *allergies*. You should take antifungal herbs: either pot marigold, chamomile, thyme, or golden seal regularly in *teas* or *tinctures*, adding echinacea to boost the immune system. *Garlic* and olive oil on salads or garlic perles will help check the infection. For oral thrush, make a *mouthwash* of thyme and pot marigold tea, allow to cool and add 1 drop of thyme or oregano oil and use 2-3 times daily. For vaginal thrush use these teas or tinctures as a douche, or soak a tampon or pad to use for an hour twice daily. Bathing in chamomile tea or applying live plain yogurt to the area can bring great relief. **Warning** Do not use douches if you are pregnant.

ME/ POST VIRAL SYNDROME

When the immune system is weakened by *stress*, poor diet, recurrent *infection*, antibiotics, or *candidiasis*, it cannot resolve an acute viral infection, which then affects other tissues, particularly the muscles and the nervous system. *Allergies* to foods, chemicals, and yeast are common. Treatment may be necessary over weeks, months, even years. Initially take, as *teas* or *tinctures*, a combination of immune-enhancing and cleansing herbs: echinacea, yellow dock root, cleavers, and wild indigo, with a little licorice to support the adrenals. Then combine with wild oats, vervain, or skullcap for the nervous system, and dandelion or barberry for the liver. You can take ginseng for three-month periods.

HERPES

The viruses of *herpes simplex* (causing cold sores and genital herpes), and *herpes zoster* (shingles), live in nerve endings, which can erupt due to poor diet, infection, and *stress*. To enhance resistance take, as *teas* or *tinctures*, a combination of echinacea, cleavers, dandelion root, and red clover, plus *garlic* 3 times daily. In shingles add St John's wort, wild oats, and skullcap to support the nervous system and relieve pain, and Jamaican dogwood if pain is extreme. You can dab teas or dilute tinctures of either golden seal, myrrh, or pot marigold on to cold sores, or use a *lotion* - 10 drops of lavender tincture, thyme or tea tree *oil* mixed with 2tsp of lavender tincture and 4tsp of water - 2-3 times daily. For shingles blisters, St John's wort and pot marigold tea or 10 drops of lavender oil in 4tsp of aqueous *cream* will help relieve pain and irritation.

Quantities: See pages 15-19

Yellow dock root (Rumex crispus) *The root is used and the* **actions** *are: gentle laxative, bitter tonic, stimulates bile production, alterative, and anti-anaemic.*

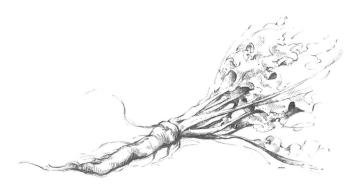

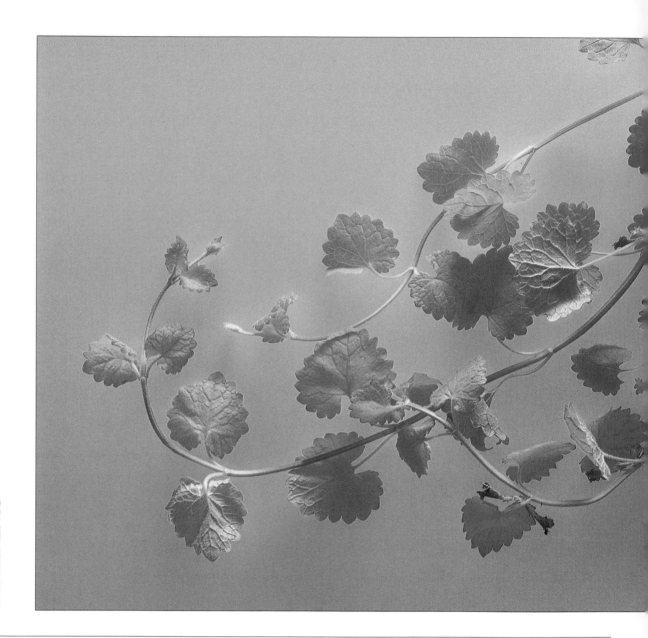

Ground ivy (Nepeta hederacea) *The aerial parts are used and the* **actions** *are: expectorant, mucous membrane tonic, antimucous/catarrhal, astringent, vulnerary, and diuretic. Ground ivy is an excellent expectorant and tonic for all mucus/catarrhal conditions,* colds *and* flu, sinusitis, *throat and chest infections, and ear problems. Its astringent properties make it valuable in* diarrhoea *and* haemorrhoids, as well as gastritis, *colitis, and* cystitis. *Externally it can be used as an inhalant for coughs, colds, and* mucus/catarrh, *as a gargle for* sore throats, *and as a* lotion *to heal wounds and ulcers. The oil is helpful massaged (see* liniment) *into painful joints, dropped into the ear in* earache, *and massaged into the head for* headaches *and* tinnitus.

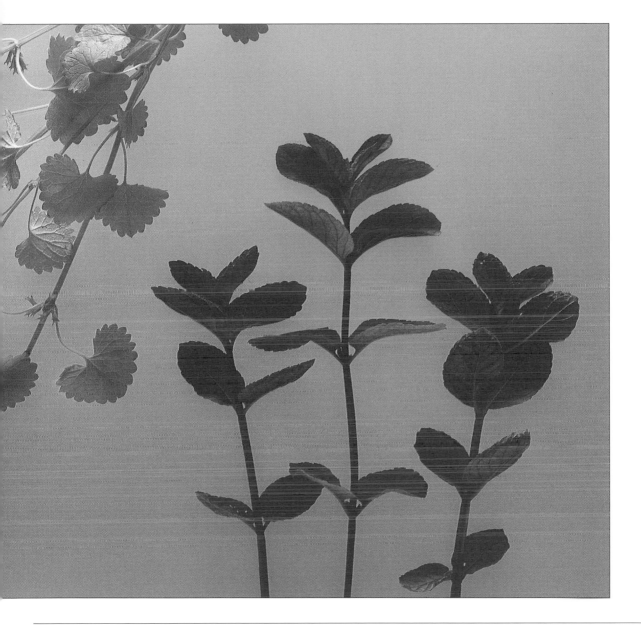

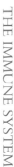

Peppermint (Mentha piperita) *The flowering herb is used, and* **actions** *are: carminative, antispasmodic, digestive, anaesthetic, anti-emetic, cholagogue, anti-inflammatory, febrifuge, antimicrobial, nerve tonic, relaxant, cooling, and circulatory stimulant. Peppermint relaxes smooth muscle in the digestive tract and reduces* colic *and* flatulence. *It relieves* nausea *and* vomiting, *stimulates secretion of digestive juices and bile, enhancing digestion, while its anti-inflammatory action is useful for ulcerative colitis and peptic ulcers. It reduces* fevers *and is valuable in respiratory infections and* mucus/catarrh. *It also acts as a nerve tonic, relieving anxiety and tension, and easing* painful periods, headaches, *and* migraines. **Warning** *Avoid prolonged use of the oil as an inhalant and never use it for babies.*

THE NERVOUS SYSTEM

Stress is a natural response to pressure, and seen positively it can bring out the best in us, provided that it is interspersed with periods of calm. Our resistance to stress can be impaired through trauma, long-term stress, chronic or frequent illness, nutritional deficiencies (see pp.26-9), allergies, and digestive problems. During periods of stress our bodies use up nutrients faster than normal, and unless these are replaced our nervous systems become progressively depleted, further reducing resistance, and thus creating a vicious circle. During times of pressure, to boost the nervous system, increase essential fatty acids, vitamins B, C, and E, and minerals calcium, magnesium, and zinc through diet or supplements. Avoid refined foods, sugar, and caffeine. Take tonics to support the nervous system: vervain, skullcap, wild oats, and ginseng.

TENSION, ANXIETY, AND STRESS

Tension or anxiety is a normal response to a difficult situation, which should settle once the problem is resolved. However, through extreme or long-term stress it may become habitual, though the original causes of it have passed. Stress-related physical problems may develop, such as stomach and bowel problems, *high blood pressure*, *allergies*, and skin problems. Take *teas* or *tinctures* of either vervain, skullcap, wild oats, or ginseng 3 times daily to support a depleted nervous system. Add either chamomile, limeflower, valerian, hops, or passionflower to soothe the nerves and relax tense muscles. Drink teas of lemon balm, chamomile, lavender, or limeflower instead of tea and coffee to help digestive problems and enhance resistance to infection and *allergy*. Take hot *herbal baths* and massage (see *liniment*), using relaxing essential *oils* of either lavender, rose, chamomile, or geranium. *Inhalations* of frankincense will calm and deepen breathing.

DEPRESSION

There may be a simple physical explanation for depression, e.g. hormone imbalance in *PMS/premenstrual tension* or post-natal depression, *allergy*, or nutritional deficiency (see pp.26-9). It is often related to a debilitation due to chronic illness, *stress*, or digestive problems. Take wild oats, skullcap, vervain, and ginseng daily, as *teas* or *tinctures*, to lift the spirits and replace essential nutrients.

Quantities: See pages 15-19

THE AILMENTS

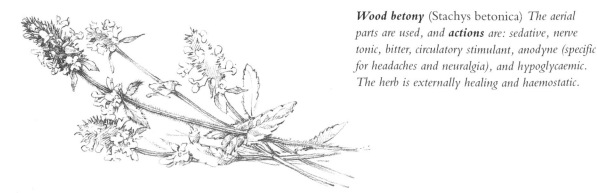

Wood betony (Stachys betonica) *The aerial parts are used, and* **actions** *are: sedative, nerve tonic, bitter, circulatory stimulant, anodyne (specific for headaches and neuralgia), and hypoglycaemic. The herb is externally healing and haemostatic.*

Drink tea made from a mixture of rosemary, vervain, dandelion, and cinnamon 3 times daily for debility and depression following illness. Add either lemon balm, damiana, borage, St John's wort, basil, or wood betony to soothe the nerves and brighten the mood. Relaxing *herbal baths* and massage (see *liniment*) with *oils* of either lavender, chamomile, bergamot, rose, or clary sage can be uplifting.

INSOMNIA

The most obvious causes are *tension, anxiety, and stress* through being run-down, over-tired, overworked, in pain, having digestive problems, *allergies, candidiasis,* nutritional deficiencies (see pp.26-9), jet lag, too much caffeine, or a lack of fresh air and exercise. A warm *herbal bath* before bed with strong *infusions* or *oils* of either limeflower, lavender, chamomile, neroli, or rose will relax tense muscles and an overactive mind. Massage (see *liniment*) is also wonderfully beneficial. Take a cup or two of *tea*, or 1-3 tsp of *tincture* of either limeflower, chamomile, catnip, lemon balm, or hops before bed (or use *sleep pillows* of these). For a persistent problem try teas or tinctures of either passionflower, valerian, or skullcap with a little licorice, and repeat if you wake. Continue nightly until you develop a good sleeping pattern and gradually reduce the dose. Take a combination of wild oats, skullcap, vervain, and rosemary as hot herbal teas 3 times daily if you are very tired and run down. Avoid all caffeine.

HEADACHES AND MIGRAINE

Headaches and migraines may be warning signs of *stress* or fatigue, but they are also related to women's hormonal problems, *allergy*, pollution, *candidiasis*, nutritional deficiency/poor diet (see pp.26-9), *high blood pressure*, low blood sugar, liver and digestive problems, alcohol, *eye strain*, and back problems. A warm *herbal bath* with strong *infusions* or *oils* of either lavender, peppermint, or marjoram will relax muscles and soothe pain. Massage (see *liniment*), particularly of the head and neck, and feet, and *inhalations* can bring swift relief. As a preventative take, either as a mixture or individually, *teas* or *tinctures* of feverfew, meadowsweet, wood betony, and rosemary 3 times daily. For *tension*, especially in the neck and shoulders, add either rosemary, valerian, or cramp bark. For menstrual problems add devil's bit/false unicorn root, or vitex. For *stress* and *anxiety* add either chamomile, vervain, skullcap, wild oats, or pasque flower. At the first signs of pain take teas or tinctures of passionflower, feverfew, rosemary, or wood betony and repeat as necessary. Inhale lavender or rosemary oils

Passionflower (Passiflora incarnata) *is mainly used as a tranquillizer. The leaves and flowers of the herb are used, and the* **actions** *are: sedative, antispasmodic, anodyne, hypotensive, and diaphoretic.*

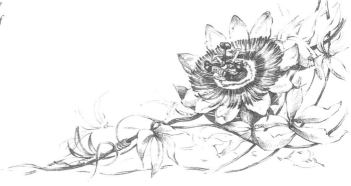

or massage them into the temples. **Warning** Headaches may indicate potentially serious, albeit uncommon, problems.

TIREDNESS AND EXHAUSTION

Your vitality may be low through chronic *stress*, *anxiety* or overwork, or *insomnia*, long-term illness, recurrent *infection*, drug therapy, poor diet (see pp. 26-9), low blood sugar, *allergy*, *candidiasis*, *anaemia*, or old age. Take, as *teas* or *tinctures*, a combination of wild oats, vervain, licorice, and skullcap to enhance recovery from *stress*. Or take bitter tonics dandelion and burdock combined with echinacea, red clover, and nettles, also as teas or tinctures, if you are run down from illness or long-term drug therapy. You may need to add a soothing digestive tonic of a mixture of slippery elm, comfrey, rosemary, and plantain to help put back essential nutrients. *Garlic* and sage aid the immune system and help fortify the nerves.

NEURALGIA

Inflammation of a nerve can cause excruciating pain. To ensure recovery the cause of the pain needs to be identified and treated by a doctor. Take a combination of ginseng, wild oats, wood betony, vervain, and licorice as *teas* or *tinctures*, if you feel tired and run down. If you feel tense and your muscles tight take, in the same way, a com-

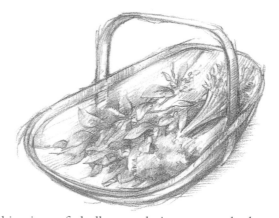

bination of skullcap, valerian, cramp bark, and wild yam and add either passionflower, black cohosh, or St John's wort if you are in a lot of pain. If the area feels hot or inflamed and there is infection (e.g. shingles) add echinacea, golden seal, and licorice. If your circulation is poor and you feel cold, angelica root and ginger will bring blood and nutrition to the area. If your bowels are sluggish, either licorice, fennel, rhubarb, or ginger will help eliminate toxins. Where there is pressure on a nerve from a spinal problem, consult a chiropractor or osteopath. Add *infusions* or dilute *oils* of either ginger, lavender, peppermint, chamomile, or rosemary to hot *herbal baths*, or you can use them for *liniments* or *compresses*. St John's wort oil specific for damaged nerves and neuralgia is wonderfully pain-relieving and can be gently massaged in (see *liniment*). **Warning** Weakness or paralysis require immediate medical attention.

Quantities: See pages 15-19

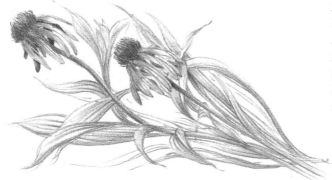

Echinacea (Echinacea angustifolia) *is also known as cone flower. The parts used are the roots and rhizomes, and the* **actions** *are: immune enhancing, antimicrobial, alterative, and externally healing to wounds, ulcers, and skin conditions. The herb is recommended for all infections, including viruses and* allergies.

THE AILMENTS

THE RESPIRATORY SYSTEM

The respiratory system is vulnerable to environmental pollution and infection, and also to an overload of internal toxins from poor diet, lack of fresh air and exercise, and congested bowels. Allergies and infections can develop when resistance is lowered by nutritional deficiencies (see pp.26-9), tiredness, stress, and frequent illness.

Breathing deeply and rhythmically is essential to our wellbeing; sufficient oxygen is necessary for healthy functioning of every cell in the body and vital for our nerves and muscles. Fresh air and exercise can help prevent respiratory ailments, and enhance our ability to deal with pain and stress. A healthy diet with plenty of vitamin C and E is essential to minimize damage to the lungs from pollution. Herbs such as garlic, thyme, and sage taken regularly will help prevent infection.

COLDS AND FLU

A virus will thrive if you are run down, stressed, lack exercise, have sluggish bowels, or are overloaded with toxins. The resulting symptoms, particularly *fever* and *mucus/catarrh*, allow the body to cleanse itself. At the first signs drink a hot *tea* made from a mixture of boneset, elderflower, peppermint, and yarrow every hour or two; this relieves aches and pains, reduces *fever* by encouraging perspiration, and clears *mucus/catarrh*. Equally effective is a delicious spicy tea made from a *decoction* of 1oz (28g) fresh ginger, 1 cinnamon stick, 1tsp coriander seeds, and 4 cloves, sweetened with honey. Frequent *inhalations* using *infusions* or *oils* of either thyme, eucalyptus, rosewood, cinnamon, or cloves will help loosen and clear the *mucus/catarrh*. A hot *foot bath* using these, or 1tbsp of mustard powder, will stimulate circulation and aid elimination of the virus. To help fight the infection take echinacea as a tea or *tincture* every 2 hours and *garlic*, raw in honey, or 2 perles, 3 times daily.

MUCUS/CATARRH AND SINUS PROBLEMS

Drink hot *teas*, either as a mixture or individually, of chamomile, peppermint, hyssop, ginger, or cinnamon to stimulate the mucous membranes and help loosen the mucus/catarrh. If it persists, add to the basic tea astringent herbs, either golden seal, eyebright, elderflower, or plantain. Demulcent herbs marshmallow and comfrey will soothe irritation and soreness. Take echinacea and

Golden seal (Hydrastis canadensis) *is a well-known North American Indian remedy. The roots and rhizome are the parts used and the* **actions** *are: tonic, astringent, antimucous/catarrhal, bitter tonic, antimicrobial, oxytocic, cholagogue, laxative, healing, and sedative.* **Warning** *Avoid taking during pregnancy.*

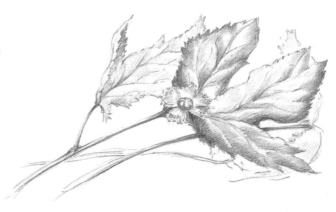

garlic to help combat infection. To relieve congestion use *infusions* or *oils* for *inhalations*, in *vaporizers*, in *herbal baths*, or for massage (see *liniment*) around the nose, sinuses, throat, or chest, using either lavender, peppermint, pine, thyme, eucalyptus, or chamomile. Mucus/catarrh and sinusitis can occur in a chronic form, with or without infection, due to irritation from pollution, or as an attempt by the body to eliminate toxins. A milk *allergy* can cause mucus/catarrh and recurrent respiratory infections. In addition to the above remedies you may need to drink licorice and dandelion root tea, or take psyllium seeds for sluggish bowels. Drink plenty of liquids such as hot lemon and honey, and teas of cleavers, chamomile, and celery seed to increase urination, and take plenty of vigorous exercise. Either yarrow, garlic, ginger, limeflower, or cinnamon in hot teas or hot foods will increase elimination of toxins through the skin, helping to relieve mucus/catarrhal congestion and infection. A humidifier may also be useful.

EARACHE

Earache can arise from pain in the throat, gums, teeth, parotid glands (in mumps), an inflammation of the outer ear canal (often caused by *eczema*, *boils*, or objects put in the ear). For this, wash discharge away with warm chamomile or pot marigold *tea*. Drop some warm olive oil with a few drops of either lavender, garlic, or chamomile *oil* into the ear and plug it with cotton ball/wool to relieve inflammation or infection.

Acute middle ear infection can cause pain and may require antibiotics (see your doctor). Provided there is no pus from a perforated eardrum (check with your doctor) you can drop a little warmed oil into the ear to help relieve pain and clear infection. Use oils of either mullein, garlic, St John's wort, or lavender diluted in olive oil. Add a few drops of golden seal or myrrh *tincture*. Take a combination of chamomile, skullcap, hyssop, and echinacea, as teas or tinctures, to aid relaxation, soothe pain, and resolve infection. Add limeflower if there is a *fever*. For recurrent ear infections or glue ear look for underlying causes such as chronic throat, tonsil, sinus, or mucus/catarrhal problems, and avoid mucus-producing foods, and note that passive smoking has been linked with glue ear. Take *garlic* daily, as well as supplements of cod liver oil and vitamin C (see p.28), and a mixture of echinacea, chamomile, licorice, elderflower, cleavers, and golden seal as teas or tinctures, to help clear *mucus/catarrh*, resolve infection and enlarged tonsils, which can block the eustachian tube. Use oils of either eucalyptus, rosewood, chamomile, or lavender for

Quantities: See pages 15-19

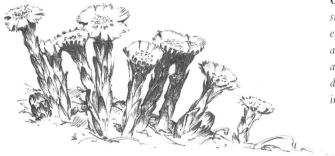

Coltsfoot (Tussilago farfara) *The Latin name signifies coltsfoot's ancient use of the herb as a remedy for coughs. The flowers and leaves are used, and* **actions** *(internally) are: soothing expectorant, antitussive, demulcent, antimucous/catarrhal, and diuretic. Externally actions are: soothing and healing to sore and inflamed skin conditions.*

inhalation and to massage (see *liniment*) around the ears and throat.

SORE THROAT

At the first signs of a sore throat *gargle* or *spray* the throat with *teas* or *tinctures* of either thyme, golden seal, or myrrh 3-6 times a day. Alternatively red sage with a teaspoon of cider vinegar can be effective, as can hot salt water, or hot water and lemon. Take antiseptic herbs, as teas or tinctures, to help the immune system: echinacea, golden seal, and sage every 2 hours, and *garlic* 3 times daily. Add to the basic mixture elderflower, yarrow, and peppermint for *mucus/catarrh*, a *fever*, or *flu*. Add soothing herbs mullein, marshmallow, or coltsfoot if the throat is particularly sore. Add cleavers or pot marigold when the neck glands are swollen or uncomfortable. Sweeten teas with licorice. Use antiseptic oils for *inhalations*, in vaporizers and for *compresses*, or massage (see *liniment*) either lavender, rosewood, chamomile, or eucalyptus around the throat.

TONSILLITIS

In acute tonsillitis use an antiseptic *gargle* or *throat spray* of sage and thyme, or chamomile and ground ivy every hour or two. Add marshmallow if the throat is very painful. Apply *compresses* of these *teas* to the throat and neck, massage (see *liniment*) dilute *oils* of either chamomile, thyme, rosewood, or lemon into the area and use them as *inhalations* or *room sprays*. To help clear the infection and soothe the throat take *garlic* and drink a hot tea made from a mixture of chamomile, ground ivy, mullein, pot marigold, and echinacea every hour or two, alternated with hot lemon and honey drinks. Continue until all infection has cleared. For chronic or recurrent bouts, drink a tea made from a mixture of echinacea, pot marigold, nettles, chamomile, and burdock to raise resistance and help clear out toxins. Use gargles or throat sprays of sage and thyme tea, or dilute *tincture* of either myrrh, sage, or golden seal, and massage dilute oils of either lavender, eucalyptus, or chamomile into the throat night and morning. Take garlic 3 times daily. **Warning** See your doctor if your child has a *fever* with tonsillitis so that streptococcal tonsillitis can be ruled out.

LARYNGITIS AND PHARYNGITIS

Steam *inhalations* are very soothing, using anti-inflammatory and antiseptic *oils* of either rosewood, lavender, sandalwood, or chamomile, and can bring swift relief. Use the same oils for massage (see *liniment*), or *infusions* of either mullein, sage, thyme, or hyssop for *compresses* applied around the throat and chest. Use sage and thyme *tea*, or dilute *tincture* of myrrh or golden seal for *gar-*

THE RESPIRATORY SYSTEM

Elecampane (Inula helenium) *The Latin name comes from Helen of Troy, from whose tears the herb is said to have sprung. The parts used are the root and rhizome, and the **actions** are: antiseptic, antimicrobial (specifically for chest infections), warming expectorant, bitter tonic, cholagogue, anthelmintic, diaphoretic, and digestive.*

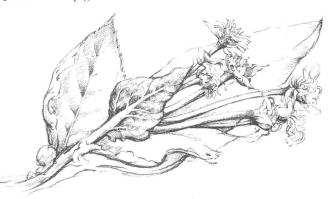

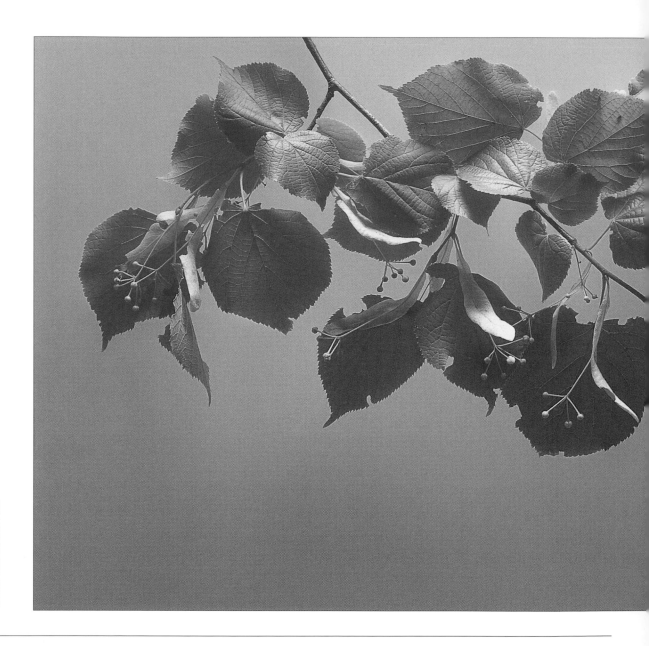

Limeflower (Tilia europaea) *The flowers are used and the* **actions** *are: diaphoretic, febrifuge, relaxant, hypotensive, mild astringent, diuretic, and antispasmodic. In hot infusion limeflower induces sweating and reduces* fevers, *and is therefore a useful treatment for* colds, flu, *and childhood infectious diseases. It also relaxes the nervous system, so is used to ease* tension, anxiety, *and* insomnia. *It reduces* high blood pressure, *especially in nervous* tension *and helps prevent arteriosclerosis. It is also helpful in nervous* headaches, *digestive problems of nervous origin,* palpitations, *and dizziness. Its mild astringent properties make it useful for* mucous/catarrh *and* diarrhoea, *while its diuretic action is useful in* water retention *and* cystitis.

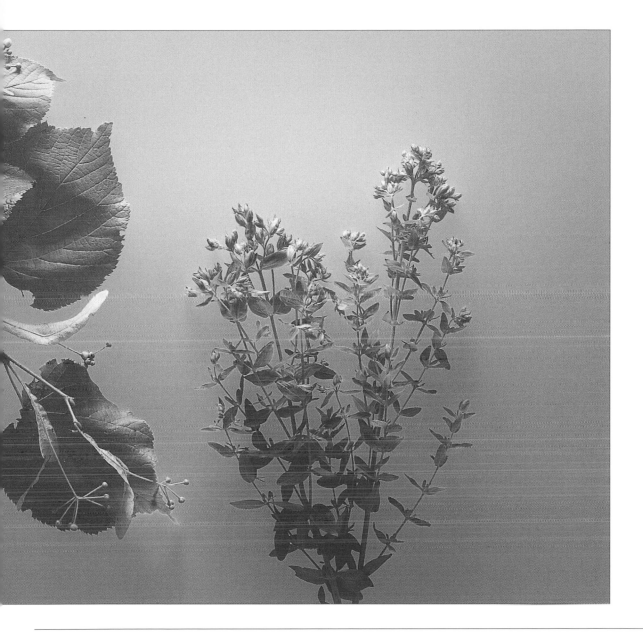

St John's wort (Hypericum perforatum) *The aerial parts are used and* **actions** *are: anti-inflammatory, astringent, vulnerary, sedative, relaxant, anodyne, antidepressant, diuretic, expectorant, antispasmodic, and antiseptic. Internally St John's wort is relaxing, sedative, and pain killing, helpful for* anxiety, tension, *and* neuralgia, *and useful for menopausal anxiety, irritability, or depression. Its diuretic action helps* arthritis *and* gout *and it is used as an expectorant for coughs and* bronchitis, *and as an anti-inflammatory remedy in* gastritis *and stomach* ulcers. *Externally it has a wide reputation for healing* cuts, burns, *and* wounds. *The oil is excellent for* neuralgia, *sciatic pain, fibrositis, and rheumatic pain.* **Warning** *Can cause sensitivity to sunlight. Avoid prolonged use.*

gles or *throat sprays* 3-6 times daily. Drink teas made from a mixture of echinacea, mullein, catnip, coltsfoot, and thyme, flavoured with licorice, every 2 hours, and *garlic* 3 times daily. Add fennel or black co-hosh to the tea if you have a painful, tight *cough*, and either yarrow, limeflower, or el-derflower if you have a *fever*. Alternate with hot lemon and honey drinks or blackcurrant tea. Keep room air moist with *room sprays* of tea or oils of either pine, eucalyptus, birch leaves, or lavender diluted in water.

ASTHMA

An asthma attack can be triggered by: an al-lergic reaction to dietary or environmental allergens, irritation (e.g from smoky, cold, or foggy atmospheres), a respiratory infec-tion, emotional problems, or digestive disturbance. Prevention is the best line of treatment. You can use herbs in conjunction with other medication or inhalants, how-ever, you may need to take them over several months. Take *garlic* regularly, and *teas* or *tinctures* of echinacea, licorice, and borage to support the immune system and adrenal glands and combine them with coltsfoot, hyssop, elecampane, and thyme to strengthen the lungs, relax the bronchial tubes and help expel *mucus/catarrh*. If you feel tense add either skullcap, vervain, or chamomile. If you suffer from profuse mucus/catarrh add golden seal and tea of el-derflower and peppermint. In an acute attack use hot *foot baths* and apply *compresses* frequently to the chest (made with tea of a mixture of thyme, coltsfoot, hyssop, and licorice). Take a tea made from equal parts of coltsfoot, chamomile, thyme, elecam-pane, and borage and half parts of ginger and licorice, every ¼-1 hour. Thyme tea alone is beneficial if your attack is mild. At the first signs of a *cold* or *cough* treat vigorously as res-piratory infections invariably make asthma worse. **Warning** Consult your doctor if you have an attack.

HAY FEVER AND RHINITIS

If you suffer from hay fever take herbs for the immune system: ginseng and echinacea as *teas* or *tinctures*, and *garlic*, for a few months before the hay fever season starts. And take 1-2 dessertspoonsful of local honey in honeycombs with each meal for 2-4 months beforehand. Continue with both of these through the season. Once the season begins, omit wheat from the diet and drink teas made from a mixture of eyebright, echi-nacea, chamomile, and elderflower flavoured with licorice, as frequently as nec-essary. Take garlic every 2 hours. Steam *inhalations* of either chamomile, lemon balm, or yarrow will help relieve the congestion and calm down the allergic response. If the

Quantities: See pages 15-19

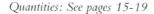

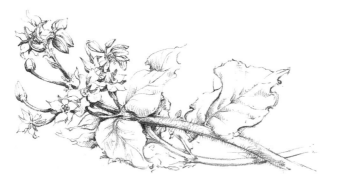

Borage (Borago officinalis) *is a herb that merits further medical investigation. The leaves, flowers, and seeds are used, and the* **actions** *are: diaphoretic, febrifuge, expectorant, tonic, anti-in-flammatory, galactagogue, and antidepressant. Borage is supportive and restorative to the adrenal glands.* **Warning** *Avoid prolonged use.*

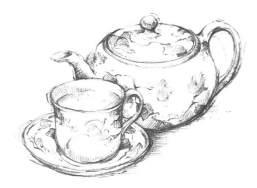

mucus/catarrh is particularly persistent, use teas or *oils* of ginger or cinnamon. For rhinitis that persists all year stop eating dairy produce and take teas or tinctures of golden seal, eyebright, elderflower, and chamomile, flavoured with licorice, as well as garlic and echinacea 3 times daily. Use teas or oils of either chamomile, lemon balm, pine, or lavender for soothing and relaxing *herbal baths* and inhalations.

COUGHS AND BRONCHITIS

A cough is a reflex response to remove anything blocking the throat or bronchial tubes. You can use herbs to help clear the chest of irritation, phlegm, and infection and to enhance the efforts of the immune system. For a dry, irritating cough take soothing herbs: either marshmallow, coltsfoot, mullein, or comfrey, as *teas* or *tinctures*, all of which can be flavoured with licorice or fennel. Once the cough has loosened and is producing phlegm drink hot teas of expectorant herbs, either as a mixture or individually, elecampane, hyssop, and thyme. If you have copious *mucus/catarrh* add ginger and cinnamon, which are warming and stimulating. If you have *fever* and malaise with the cough, or green phlegm, consult your doctor, for you may have acute bronchitis. Drink teas of either elderflower, yarrow, or limeflower combined with echinacea frequently through the day to bring down the *fever* and help clear the infection. For the chest take teas or tinctures of elecampane and combine it with coltsfoot, mullein, and licorice if the cough is dry, or hyssop and thyme if it is productive. Use these in *herbal baths* or use for *inhalations* or warm *compresses* to the chest. Take frequent drinks of hot lemon and honey, blackcurrant tea, and take garlic perles 3 times daily. For frequent or chronic bronchitis look for the causes of lowered vitality of the immune and respiratory systems. Smoking, poor diet (see pp.26-9), insufficient fresh air and exercise, pollution, *stress*, and *allergies* are possibilities. Take *garlic* and echinacea to enhance your immunity and teas made from a mixture of elecampane, mullein, coltsfoot, thyme, and licorice for the chest 3 times daily. Use these or *oils* of either thyme, eucalyptus, cinnamon, or pine for herbal baths and inhalations. **Warning** If a cough is persistent, seek medical attention.

Quantities: See pages 15-19

Mullein (Verbascum thapsus) *The flowers and leaves are used, and **actions** are: soothing expectorant, sedative, diuretic, demulcent, vulnerary, anodyne, and antispasmodic.*

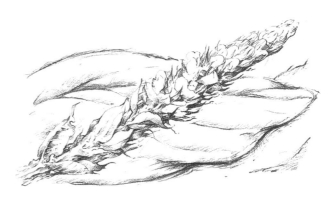

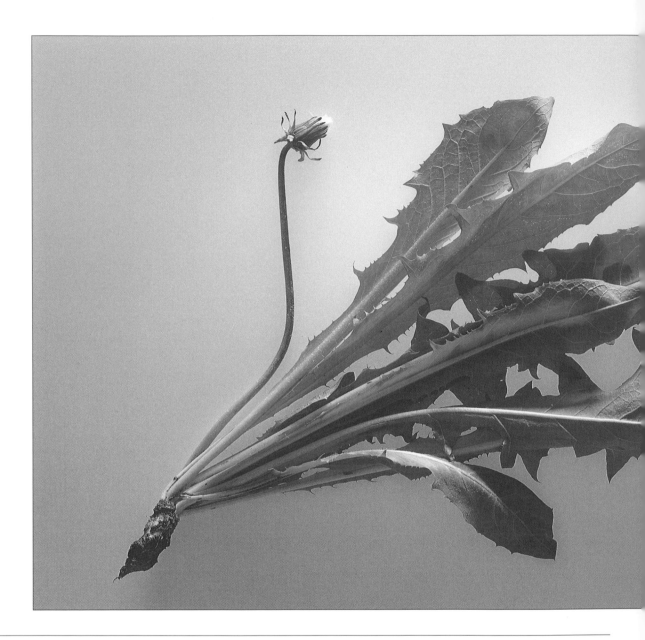

Dandelion (Taraxacum officinale) *The roots and leaves are the parts used and the* **actions** *are: (root) bitter tonic, antirheumatic, cholagogue, laxative, nutritive, alterative; (leaves) diuretic and bitter tonic. The root stimulates both the liver and gallbladder, making it a valuable remedy for* constipation, dyspepsia, and liver and gallbladder disease. *It is useful as a general tonic and can be included in treatments* for arthritis, *skin disease, digestive insufficiency, and convalescence. The leaves act as a powerful diuretic and are rich in potassium. The whole plant is a valuable nutritive alterative, cleansing the blood and tissues. Externally the sap from the stem has a reputation for removing* warts.

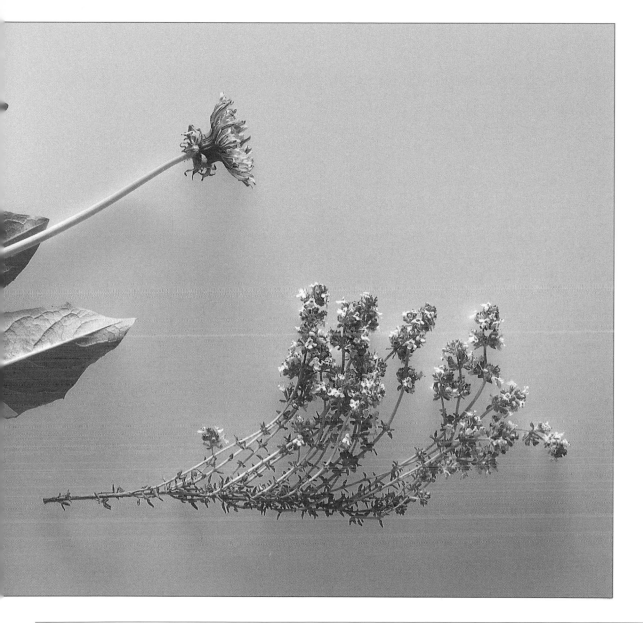

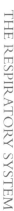
Thyme (Thymus vulgaris) *The leaves and flowering tops are used and the* **actions** *are: antibacterial, antifungal, anthelmintic, expectorant, febrifuge, diaphoretic, astringent, carminative, nerve and circulatory tonic, diuretic, antispasmodic. Thyme has powerful antibacterial and antifungal properties, which can also expel worms. It can be used for respiratory and digestive infections; it works well as a gargle or* mouthwash *for* sore throats, laryngitis, *and* tonsillitis, *and for infected gums. Its expectorant action is valuable for irritable* coughs, bronchitis, whooping cough, *and* asthma. *In hot infusion thyme induces sweat, reduces* fevers, *and relieves* colds *and* catarrh. *As a gentle astringent it relieves* diarrhoea, *and also reduces* indigestion, flatulence, *and* colic.

THE DIGESTIVE SYSTEM

The digestive tract is a long, hollow, muscular factory processing the food we eat into the substances and energy we need to keep us alive and healthy. For efficient digestion we need to eat the right foods (see pp.26-9), with plenty of fibre, to ensure regular evacuation of food residues and waste products. Junk foods, too much sugar, fatty foods, meat, alcohol, and tobacco, as well as wrong food combinations, can all irritate and disturb digestion. Stress is one of the major factors disturbing blood and nerve supply to the gut and upsetting stomach acid production, causing a wide range of digestive problems such as indigestion, ulcers, and an irritable bowel.

CONSTIPATION

Eating too much refined food and not enough fruit, vegetables, and whole grains is a major cause of constipation. Liver problems, dietary deficiency (see pp.26-9), lack of exercise, food *allergy*, and *stress* can also be to blame. With ageing our bowel muscles become weaker and bowel function sluggish, aggravated by long-term use of laxatives. Gentle remedies linseed or psyllium seeds will bulk out bowel contents and help push them along. Soak 1-2tsp of seeds in a cup of hot water for 2 hours. Add lemon and honey and drink at bedtime; if the problem persists have the drink in the morning as well. If necessary take more stimulating laxative herbs for a week or two – a *decoction* of licorice, ginger, dandelion root, yellow dock root, and burdock 3 times daily. If you feel tense add either chamo-

mile, hops, or cramp bark. **Warning** If your problem persists or you develop sudden or painful constipation, consult your doctor.

DIARRHOEA

Acute diarrhoea represents the body's attempt to rid itself of poisons or irritants, inflammation, or infection in the gut. It can also be due to faulty diet (see pp.26-9) and *stress*. For mild diarrhoea take meadowsweet frequently, as a *tea* or *tincture*, to soothe and tone the gut. If it is more severe take either agrimony, cinnamon, marshmallow, raspberry, or blackberry leaves. Add either ginger, peppermint, or chamomile for cramping pain. Arrowroot is also very effective. Mix 1tbsp arrowroot to a smooth paste with a little water. Add 1pt/600ml boiling water, stirring to thicken. Flavour with honey, lemon, or cinnamon. If you have an

Quantities: See pages 15-19

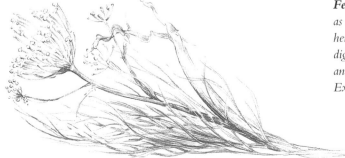

Fennel (Foeniculum vulgare) *root has been used as a vegetable and medicine since ancient times. In herbalism the seeds are used and the* **actions** *are: digestive, antispasmodic, carminative, galactagogue, antibacterial, diuretic, stimulant, and expectorant. Externally it can be used as a rubefacient.*

infection take teas or tinctures of chamomile, thyme, ginger, and fennel either individually or in combination, and garlic perles every 2 hours. If you feel tense add more chamomile, lemon balm, or wild yam to help relax the gut. **Warning** If the attack persists (for over 24 hours in a baby) or is accompanied by *fever*, or there is mucus or blood in the stools, consult your doctor.

NAUSEA AND VOMITING

Nausea and vomiting can be due to an adverse reaction to foods or drugs, nervous *tension, migraine*, or infections causing irritation and inflammation of the gut, often coupled with *diarrhoea*. To help settle the stomach sip *teas* of either ginger, chamomile, fennel, or peppermint *slowly*. If you feel nervous or tense take teas or *tinctures* of either lemon balm, hops, or passionflower, and if you have infection or food poisoning take *garlic* every 2 hours and add lemon juice to water or teas. Drink teas made from a mixture of lavender, lemon balm, and thyme with drops of echinacea or golden seal. Honey water spiced with ginger or cinnamon is delicious and particularly good for children. To treat an accompanying *fever* take either limeflower, yarrow, or elderflower as teas or tinctures. **Warning** If symptoms persist or there is severe vomiting with a high *fever* call your doctor.

HEARTBURN AND INDIGESTION

These are symptoms of a disordered stomach, often of a gastro-esophageal reflux and *hyperactivity*, caused by chronic *constipation*, obesity or *stress*, and triggered by upset or excitement, too much rich, fatty, or spicy food, alcohol, tea, coffee, or cigarettes. The underlying cause needs to be treated for there to be effective relief. At the first twinge of discomfort take slippery elm tablets. Drink *tea* made from a mixture of meadowsweet, comfrey, marshmallow, and licorice, and teas of either chamomile, fennel, peppermint, or rosemary after a meal to help digestion and settle the stomach. Take *decoctions* of dandelion and burdock as aperitifs to enhance digestion and prevent indigestion. If you are tense add either chamomile, hops, or lemon balm.

DIVERTICULITIS

Diverticulitis may develop as a result of lack of exercise, an over-refined diet (see pp.26-9), and long-term *constipation*. Infection and inflammation may cause cramping pains and irregular bowel movements. Avoid any indigestible foods (i.e. seeds, nuts, fruit skins, raw vegetables, excess roughage) until the pain subsides. Then eat a high-fibre diet, but no bran. Take a combination of wild yam, chamomile, ginger, licorice, marshmallow, and peppermint as *teas* or *tinctures* 3 times

---

Quantities: See pages 15-19

Ginseng (Panax ginseng) *In Chinese "Renshen", meaning "man root" is the king of tonics. The root is used and the **actions** are: adaptogenic, both sedative and stimulating on the central nervous system. Ginseng increases resistance to mental and physical stress, and is antidepressive and a tonic for old age or debility.*

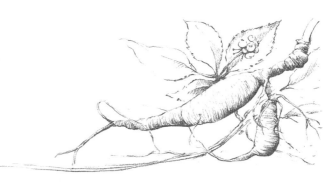

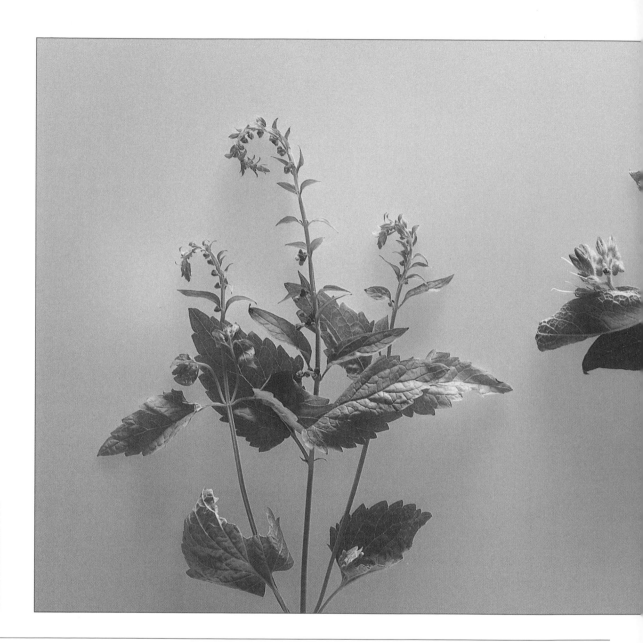

Skullcap (Scutellaria laterifolia) *The aerial parts of the herb are used and the* **actions** *are: nerve tonic, relaxant, antidepressant, analgesic, digestive, sedative, and antispasmodic. Skullcap is a wonderful tonic to the nervous system, helpful in easing anxiety, and tension, depression, insomnia, exhaustion, and nervous headaches. It relaxes tension while at the same time revitalizing and supporting a debilitated nervous system. Skullcap has an ancient reputation for treating hysteria and epilepsy. It strengthens the digestive system, and relieves premenstrual tension, neuralgia, and rheumatic pain.*

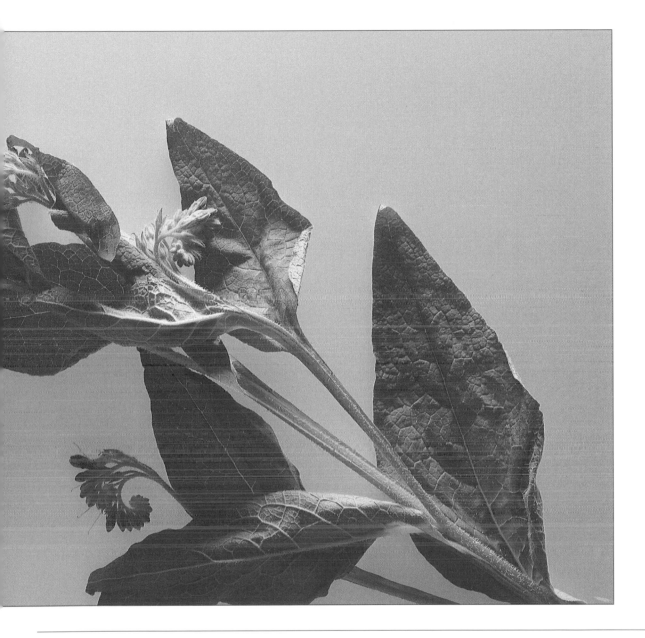

Comfrey (Symphytum officinale) *The roots and leaves are the parts used and the **actions** are: vulnerary, emollient, demulcent, cell-proliferator, soothing expectorant, diuretic, ovarian tonic, reputed anti-cancer action, and astringent. This famous herb is renowned for its ability to heal bones and tissues, due to the presence of allantoin, a constituent stimulating active cell growth. It can speed the healing of* cuts and wounds, *and it also heals ulcers, fractures,* burns, and bruises. *Internally the presence of soothing mucilage makes comfrey a valuable remedy for* peptic ulcers, gastritis and ulcerative colitis. *Comfrey is also a soothing expectorant, useful for* bronchitis and irritable coughs. *It is also a soothing remedy for the urinary system.*

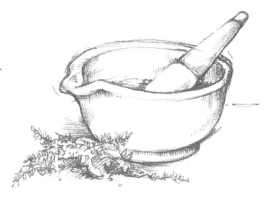

daily with meals to relax and heal the gut. Take *garlic* 3 times daily to counter the bacteria that fill the diverticuli, and 1 cupful of slippery elm *gruel* 3 times daily to help heal the bowel wall. Take 1tsp of linseed or psyllium seeds expanded in a cup of water once or twice daily to regulate the bowels and prevent either *diarrhoea* or *constipation*.

IRRITABLE BOWEL SYNDROME AND SPASTIC COLITIS

The lining of the bowel is particularly susceptible to the effects of *stress*, as well as bad eating habits (see pp.26-9), and food intolerance, and may become irritated, leading to irritable bowel syndrome or spastic colitis. The bowel becomes overactive with alternating *diarrhoea* and *constipation*, *flatulence*, and discomfort. Food intolerance is frequently at the root of the problem, so you may need to temporarily omit foods such as tea, coffee, milk products, eggs, wheat, or gluten while you take herbs to treat the bowel. Take, as *teas* or *tinctures*, a combination of wild yam, chamomile, peppermint, agrimony, marshmallow, and golden seal 3-6 times daily to soothe the bowel and resolve the inflammation. Add hops and more chamomile for *stress*, and more marshmallow for pain. Take slippery elm *gruel* with a pinch of cinnamon or ginger powder as required. **Warning** If there is much mucus or

blood in your stools or you experience severe abdominal pain, see your doctor.

FLATULENCE

Bloating and gas/wind are a symptom of a variety of digestive disturbances and you need a clear diagnosis for the cause to be treated effectively. Common causes are: unconsciously swallowing air, particularly when nervous, weak digestion, and bad eating habits. *Gastritis*, *gallbladder disease*, *peptic ulcer*, food *allergies*, *candidiasis*, *constipation*, *irritable bowel*, and *stress* can also be to blame. Carminative herbs are specific for relieving gas/wind, the best of which are wild yam, peppermint, ginger, cinnamon, fennel, lemon balm, and chamomile taken as *teas*, or a few drops of *tincture* in warm water after meals. Warming spices added to your cooking, such as cayenne, ginger, cardamon, and caraway seeds are also helpful. Gentle massage (see *liniment*) of the abdomen

THE AILMENTS

52

Quantities: See pages 15-19

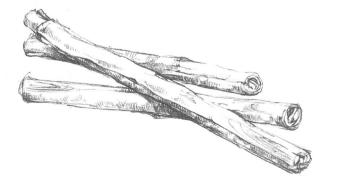

Cinnamon (Cinnamomum zeylanicum) *has been valued as a medicine to treat* colds *and* flu, *to warm the digestion, and to ease* flatulence, *since ancient times. The dried bark is used, and the* **actions** *are: carminative, warming to the digestive tract, astringent, and antispasmodic. The oil is antibacterial and antifungal, used for treating thrush.*

(clockwise) using dilute *oils* of either cinnamon, ginger, cloves, or peppermint can be very effective.

GASTRITIS AND PEPTIC ULCERS

The stomach may become irritated and inflamed through weak digestion, bad eating habits (see pp.26-9), and *stress*, causing gastritis. As the condition worsens, ulceration of the gut lining can develop. The herbal approach aims to resolve the inflammation and heal the damaged lining while relieving *tension* and *stress*. The first choice is chamomile, either taken as a strong *tea* (double the normal dose) or ½ tsp *tincture* in a glass of warm water on an empty stomach 4 times a day. Other useful remedies, also taken as teas or tinctures, include licorice, marshmallow, comfrey, meadowsweet, golden seal, and pot marigold. Slippery elm *gruel* taken as required will provide quick relief from pain and, by coating the gut lining, protects it from irritation and acidity. If you are feeling particularly stressed or tense add relaxants and nerve tonics of either hops, lemon balm, vervain or skullcap, and use *oils* of either lavender, chamomile, or lemon balm in *herbal baths* and for massage (see *liniment*). Eat little and often and avoid rich, fatty food, pickles, alcohol, tobacco, tea, and coffee as much as possible. **Warning** Acute abdominal pain, with a known history of ulcers, may indicate perforation and requires immediate medical attention.

GALLSTONES AND GALLBLADDER PROBLEMS

Gallstones can form in the gallbladder from excessive concentration of bile contents, notably cholesterol, and cause great pain. The gallbladder can become infected or inflamed, producing *indigestion*, stomach and gallbladder pain, especially after eating fatty foods. For acute biliary colic and inflammation take, as *teas* or *tinctures*, a mixture of dandelion root, wild yam, fumitory, lemon balm, peppermint, and licorice every hour or two until the pain subsides. Add a mixture of valerian, fennel, and chamomile if pain is intense. For chronic, intermittent pain provoked by eating especially fatty foods, take, either as a tea or a tincture, a mixture of agrimony, yarrow, dandelion root, fumitory, peppermint, wild yam, and greater celandine 3 times daily. Dandelion root is especially recommended where there is a tendency to form stones, when it should be combined with greater celandine, chamomile, wild yam, marshmallow, and peppermint. Slippery elm *gruel* and licorice are also useful. **Warning** Development of jaundice (yellow skin colour or eyes) may indicate obstruction by a gallstone and requires medical intervention.

Quantities: See pages 15-19

Greater celandine (Chelidonium majus) *The aerial parts are used, and* **actions** *are: cholagogue, bitter, antispasmodic, anodyne, purgative, narcotic, reputed anticancer agent. Externally the orange latex is used for* warts, verrucae, *skin tumours, and tinea (ringworm).* **Warning** *Greater celandine is poisonous in large doses.*

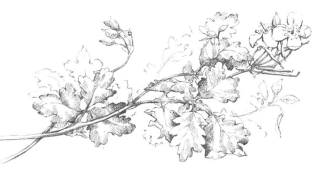

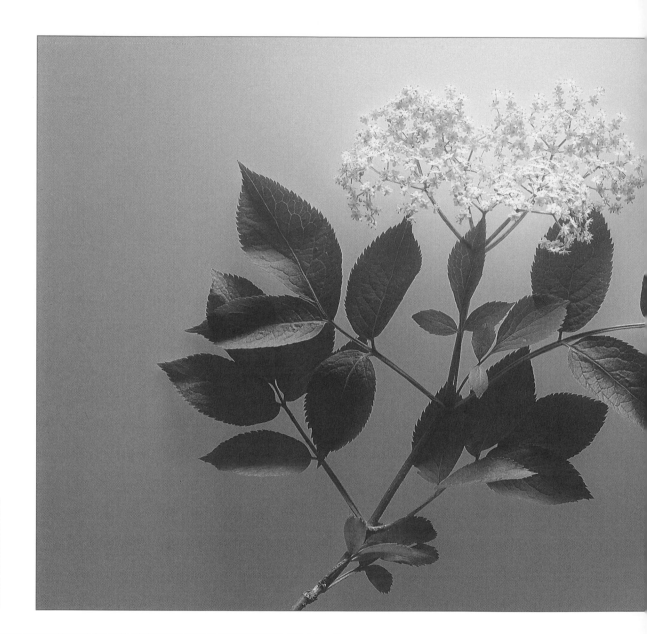

Elderflower (Sambucus nigra) *Both the flowers and berries are used, and the* **actions** *are: astringent, antimucous/catarrhal, febrifuge, circulatory stimulant, laxative, diuretic, and emollient. Elderflower is an excellent remedy for* colds *and* flu, mucous/catarrh, *and* fevers, *when taken in hot* infusion. Hay fever, rhinitis, *sinusitis, bronchial mucus/catarrh and mucous/catarrhal deafness also respond well. A cold* infusion *can be used as an* eyewash *for* conjunctivitis, *in a compress for* chilblains, *and as a* gargle *for* sore throats. *In an* ointment *elderflower relieves* skin irritation. *It can stimulate the circulation, is mildly laxative, and can relieve* arthritis *and* gout. *The berries are mildly laxative and diaphoretic, making a useful winter tonic for* colds, coughs, *and* flu.

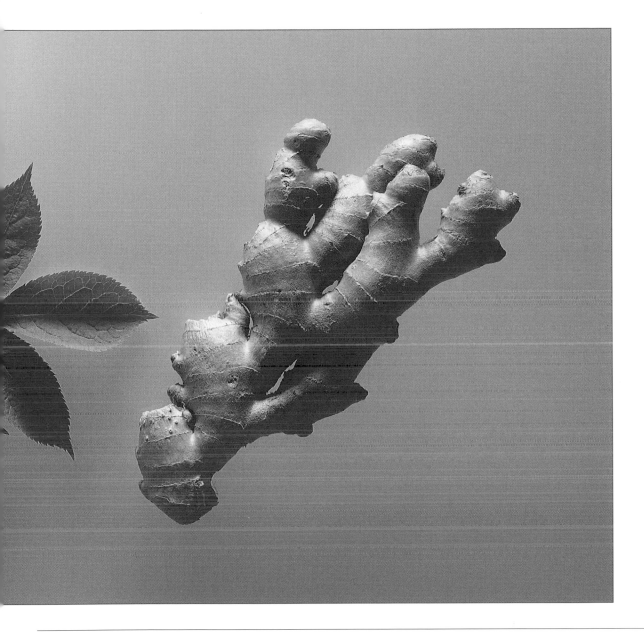

Ginger (Zinziber officinale) *The root is used and the actions are: warming, circulatory stimulant, digestive, antispasmodic, carminative, anti-emetic, diaphoretic, expectorant, and rubefacient. Ginger has a warming effect, and is beneficial in all conditions related to poor circulation, chilblains, cramp, weak digestion, and cold extremities, whether taken internally or used in* hand and foot baths. *It also relieves* colic, flatulence, *and* indigestion, morning *and* travel sickness. *It has diaphoretic properties when taken hot and is useful for feverish conditions,* colds and flu. *As a gargle it relieves* sore throats. *It also has an expectorant action, dispelling* mucus/catarrh *and* coughs. *Externally it can be used as a compress or liniment for strains and sprains, fibrositis, and aching muscles.*

THE URINARY SYSTEM

The urinary system performs the vital task of producing and excreting urine, thereby cleansing the body of waste products and helping to maintain a constant internal environment by controlling the water and chemical composition of the body. It is important to drink plenty to help the kidneys flush through toxins and prevent them from causing irritation, but avoid excess tea, coffee, alcohol, and cigarettes. During cleansing treatment use diuretic herbs, such as dandelion leaves, cleavers, and celery seed to enhance the eliminative work of the kidneys.

CYSTITIS AND URETHRITIS

Take demulcent herbs marshmallow and couch grass either as *teas* or *tinctures*, to relieve the pain and add yarrow, chamomile, or celery seed to fight the infection. If the burning is strong sit in a *herbal bath* of strong chamomile tea. Drink plenty of water, adding 1tsp baking soda (not if you have heart problems) twice daily to alkalize the urine. You can also drink soothing barley water through the day (simmer 4oz/113g washed barley in 1pt/600ml of water until the barley is soft. Add a little lemon and honey and drink luke warm). **Warning** You may need medical attention.

KIDNEY INFECTIONS AND STONES

Drink plenty and take luke warm *teas* of a mixture of echinacea, celery seed, couch grass, and buchu frequently. For stones drink 4-6pts (2-3½ litres) daily and take a combination of couch grass, dandelion leaves, cleavers, marshmallow, and stone root as *teas* or *tinctures* to help dissolve and wash out the stones and gravel. **Warning** If you think you have a kidney infection or stone, see your doctor.

WATER RETENTION

To increase excretion of water, drink lukewarm-to-cool *teas* of a mixture of dandelion leaves, celery seed, and yarrow. Add vitex or devil's bit/false unicorn root for hormonal imbalance. Avoid tea, coffee, and alcohol. Try a juice fast for 2-3 days using either celery, beetroot, watercress, watermelon, or asparagus juice for cellulite. **Warning** Water retention may indicate a serious disease - see your doctor.

Quantities: See pages 15-19

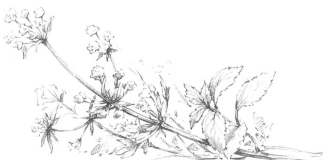

Celery seed (Apium graveolens) *The **actions** of the seeds are: diuretic, antirheumatic, urinary antiseptic, carminative, and digestive tonic, galactagogue, emmenagogue, and sedative.*
Warning *Excessive doses in pregnancy can stimulate uterine contractions.*

THE AILMENTS

THE CIRCULATORY SYSTEM

This vital transport system carries nutrients to, and waste products from, every cell and tissue in the body. We need to take great care of our heart and blood vessels by eating a healthy diet (see pp.26-9), taking regular exercise and cutting down on fats, sugar, alcohol, and smoking. Stress can play a major part in circulatory disease so it is worth considering ways of increasing your ability to deal with it, for example, by relaxation, meditation, or psychotherapy. Hawthorn and garlic are the best tonics to take as preventative measures for the heart and circulation.

ANAEMIA

It is important to establish the reason for your anaemia so that you can treat it properly. Make sure your diet (see pp.26-9) is rich in iron, folic acid, protein, and vitamin B12, and add parsley, watercress, dandelion leaves, chickweed, chives, nettles, and coriander leaves to your salads and garnishes. *Tension* and impaired digestion, tea, coffee, and too much fibre in the diet can all reduce iron absorption - you can improve this by taking *teas* or *tinctures* of iron-rich digestives burdock, yellow dock root, verbena, hawthorn, skullcap, raspberry leaves, and hops. Eat plenty of vitamin-C-rich foods (see p.28) to enhance iron absorption, and stop drinking tea and coffee.

POOR CIRCULATION AND CHILBLAINS

Take plenty of exercise and eat plenty of green, leafy vegetables. Add warming spices cayenne, ginger, coriander seeds, cloves, and cinnamon regularly to your cooking. Drink hot *teas* made from a combination of ginger, cinnamon, prickly ash, and angelica to stimulate circulation and combine them with either yarrow, hawthorn, elderflower, or peppermint to dilate the peripheral blood vessels. *Garlic*, vitamin C and bioflavonoids (see p.28), buckwheat tea, and rutin tablets are also useful. Add warming *oils* to *herbal baths* or use ginger, cinnamon, marjoram, thyme, peppermint, or rosemary oils for massage (see *liniment*). For chilblains (sores caused by exposure to cold) follow the advice above, but double the frequency. Soothe the irritation with either pot marigold/calendula *ointment*, oil of lavender, neat lemon juice, arnica ointment (not when the skin is broken), or cayenne ointment. Hot *foot baths* with oils of either marjoram, ginger, black pepper, thyme, or rosemary can be wonderfully warming.

Valerian (Valeriana officinalis) *The root is used, and* **actions** *are: sedative, antispasmodic, hypotensive, carminative, and cardiac tonic.*
Warning *Avoid large doses and prolonged use.*

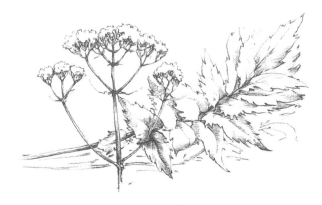

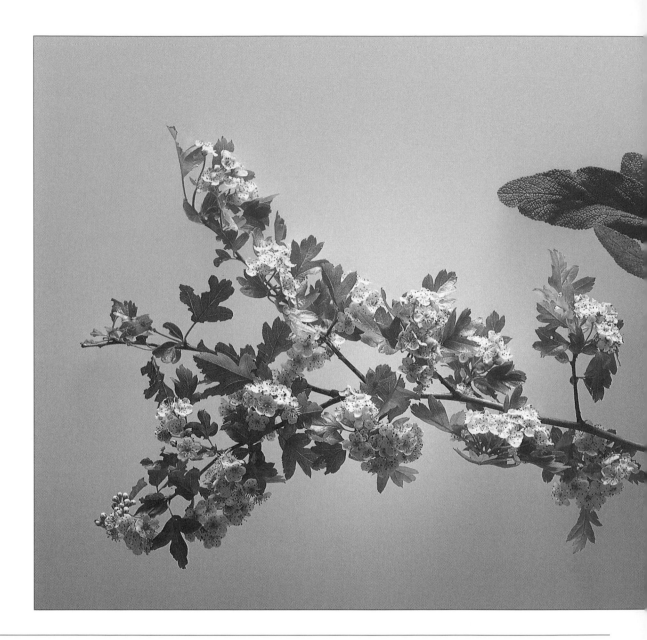

58

Hawthorn (Crataegus oxyacantha) *The parts used are the flowers, leaves, and berries. Hawthorn is a remarkable remedy for the heart and circulation. Its ability to dilate the coronary and peripheral arteries makes it valuable for use in angina,* high blood pressure, *and spasm of the arteries. It has a regulatory action on the heart, useful for irregular heartbeat and palpitations. Not only does hawthorn reduce* high blood pressure *caused by either* hardening of the arteries *or* kidney disease *but it can also be used in treatment of* low blood pressure. *It is particularly recommended as a tonic for all conditions related to an ageing heart. It also has digestive properties, useful in treatment of* diarrhoea *and* indigestion.

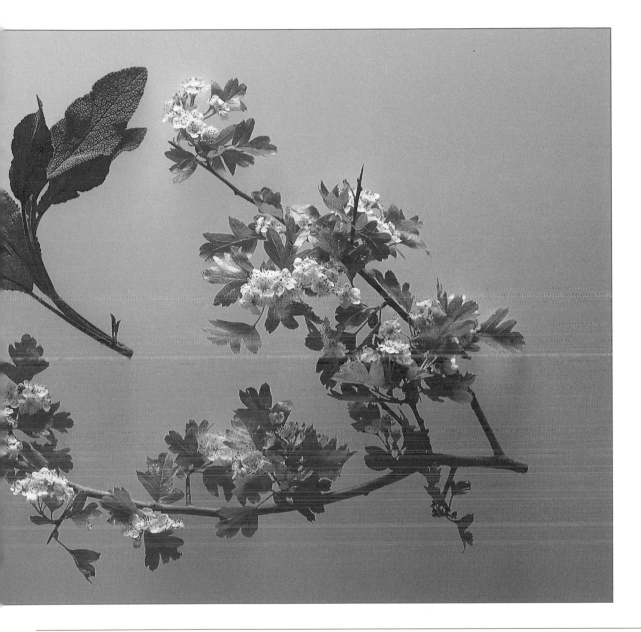

Sage (Salvia officinalis) *The leaves are used in herbalism and the* **actions** *are: antiseptic, antibacterial, carminative, digestive, oestrogenic, emmenagogue, nerve tonic, antihydrotic, antispasmodic, and astringent. Sage is an excellent antiseptic and antibacterial remedy for colds, flu, sore throats, and tonsillitis, infected gums and mouth ulcers. Its carminative and stimulating actions help colic, indigestion, and* flatulence. *Its oestrogenic action plus its ability to stop sweating helps relieve menopausal flashes/flushes. Sage can also dry up mothers' milk, and is valuable for painful periods and delayed menstruation. It strengthens the nervous system and aids convalescence.* **Warning** *Avoid during pregnancy.*

CRAMPS

Cramps are caused most commonly by *poor circulation*, *varicose veins*, chronic *tension*, tense muscles, *tiredness*, sodium and calcium imbalances, and deficiencies of vitamins B and D (see pp.26-9). Try to relax, move the limb up and down and massage it (see *liniment*) using lavender, marjoram, ginger, or rosemary *oils,* either as a mixture or individually. Hot *compresses* applied to the muscle or hot *hand and foot baths* using these oils can be rapidly effective. For poor circulation take ginger, prickly ash, and angelica as *teas* or *tinctures*, and *garlic*, and vitamin C (see p.28) regularly. To relax tense muscles take a combination of cramp bark, chamomile, skullcap, and vervain as *teas* or *tinctures*. To increase calcium intake eat parsley, watercress, sesame seeds, and dried figs, and take, as teas or tinctures, either as a combination or individually, nettles, meadowsweet, horsetail, dandelion leaves, and wild oats.

HARDENING OF THE ARTERIES

This condition can be aggravated by *high blood pressure* and by fatty infiltration of the artery walls through over-consumption of animal fats and sugar, and by alcohol, smoking, lack of exercise, and obesity. Replace all animal fats with polyunsaturated fats from cold-pressed olive, sunflower, or soya oil, oily fish, beans and pulses, and evening primrose oil and eat less fat overall even if of vegetable origin. Eat plenty of cholesterol-lowering foods such as soya beans, tofu, bran and oats, lemons, leeks and onions, and seeds. Raw *garlic* or garlic perles are especially effective. Avoid tea, coffee, alcohol, and cigarettes, and take regular exercise. Take, either as *teas* or *tinctures*, a combination of hawthorn, horsetail, limeflower, and dandelion root to improve circulation and strengthen the arteries.

HIGH AND LOW BLOOD PRESSURE

The most common causes of high blood pressure are stress, obesity, and *hardening of the arteries*. It is best to eat a vegetarian diet and take regular exercise to prevent and reduce high blood pressure. Avoid tea, coffee, alcohol, and smoking. Eat plenty of cold-pressed vegetable oils, especially olive oil, oily fish, nuts and seeds, beans and pulses, and whole grains, and take raw *garlic* or garlic perles. Take, either as *teas* or *tinctures*, a combination of hawthorn, limeflower, nettles, and motherwort 3 times daily and, if you feel tense, add either valerian, passionflower, or skullcap. Use relaxing *oils* of lavender, rosemary, lemon balm, rose, or geranium in *herbal baths* and massage oils (see *liniment*). For excess fluid take diuretic herbs: dandelion leaves in salads and teas, with corn silk, celery seed, and cleavers. **Warning** See

Quantities: See pages 15-19

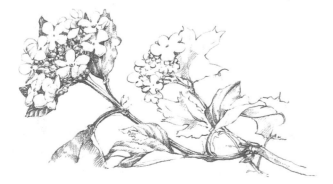

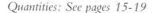

Cramp bark (Viburnum opulus) *The stem bark is used, and **actions** are: relaxant, antispasmodic, sedative, astringent with particular affinity to the pelvic area, pregnancy,* childbirth, *and menopause.*

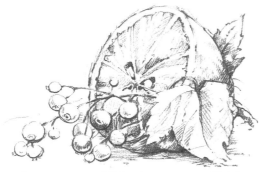

your doctor to establish the causes of high blood pressure.

For low blood pressure take ginger, cayenne, and angelica, as teas or tinctures, to stimulate the circulation; add hawthorn and nettles to help regulate the blood pressure and tonify the system. Use warming oils – either marjoram, rosemary, ginger, or cinnamon - in herbal baths, *hand and foot baths*, and for massage.

VARICOSE VEINS AND HAEMORRHOIDS

Dilation and enlargement of the veins is caused by too much standing, not enough exercise, and a familial tendency, worsened by pregnancy, *constipation*, obesity, and shallow breathing. To relieve discomfort and tone veins bathe them with a *lotion* of either distilled witch hazel, pot marigold flowers steeped in witch hazel, or *teas* of comfrey or pot marigold. You can massage (see *liniment*)

oils of either lemon, lavender, cypress, juniper, or rosemary around the area (not over the veins) or add them to *herbal baths* to increase circulation and tone and strengthen the veins. For severe aching spray the area with cold water or apply crushed ice for a few seconds. Pilewort *ointment* is wonderfully relieving for haemorrhoids. Take, as teas or *tinctures*, a combination of yarrow, St John's wort, golden seal, limeflower, and hawthorn, as well as *garlic* to improve circulation. Take supplements (see pp.26-9) of vitamins E, C, bioflavonoids, and zinc.

VARICOSE ULCERS

Where the circulation in the legs is poor, often in association with *varicose veins*, the tissues and skin begin to break down. If the leg is knocked the skin will break easily and become ulcerated. Healing can be speeded up using comfrey and honey *poultices* alternated night and morning to draw out toxins and relieve pain and inflammation. Bathe the area with pot marigold *tea* in between dressings, and dust powdered slippery elm, comfrey, or clay over the area. Take, either as teas or *tinctures*, a combination of yarrow, St John's wort, golden seal, and hawthorn regularly to help venous circulation. If an ulcer is infected or inflamed add cleavers, echinacea, and pot marigold. You may need to see a doctor.

Hops (Humulus lupulus) *has been used as a medicine for at least as long as for brewing. The dried female strobiles are used and the **actions** are: relaxant, sedative, digestive, antispasmodic, antibacterial, anti-inflammatory, oestrogenic, diuretic, anodyne, and hypnotic.* ***Warning*** *Avoid taking during depressive illness.*

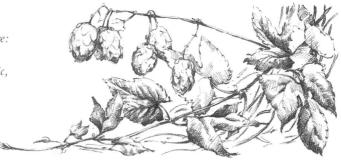

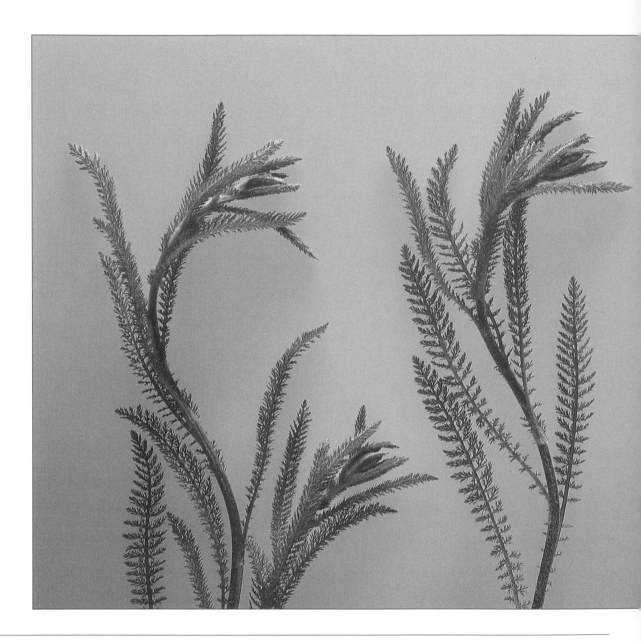

Yarrow (Achillea millefolium) *The aerial parts of the flowering plant are used, and the* **actions** *are: diaphoretic, febrifuge, peripheral vasodilator, hypotensive, antithrombotic, vulnerary, styptic, emmenagogue, anti-inflammatory, astringent, diuretic, digestive, and antiseptic.* Yarrow is a well-known remedy for fevers. *A hot* infusion *causes sweating, helping to lower a* fever *and eliminate toxins. It also lowers* blood pressure and reduces blood clots. Yarrow also acts as a digestive remedy, relieving *indigestion, gastritis, and stomach ulcers, as well as* arthritis and rheumatism. As a urinary antiseptic it is useful in *cystitis. Externally and internally it can stop bleeding, treat bleeding piles, and excessive menstrual bleeding.*

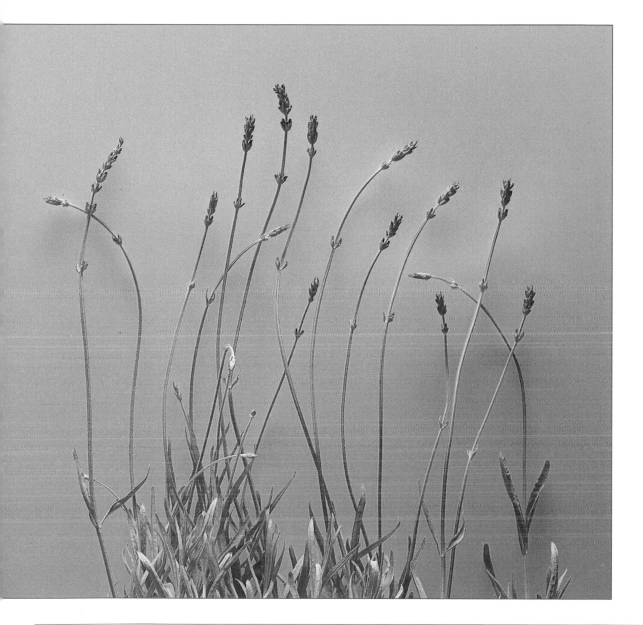

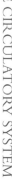

Lavender (Lavandula officinalis) *The flowers are used and* **actions** *are: relaxant, anodyne, antidepressant, nerve tonic, sedative, antimicrobial, anti-inflammatory, vulnerary, digestive, and antispasmodic. In aromatherapy lavender is used to ease* stress, tension, headaches, depression, *and to strengthen the nervous system when debilitated or exhausted. Its reported antimicrobial action is useful in all respiratory* infections. *Externally it can be used to massage painful arthritic joints and aching, tense muscles. It is also an excellent remedy for* burns, insect stings, cuts, *and* wounds. *Taken as a tea or tincture internally it has valuable antiseptic, relaxant, and digestive actions, useful in* indigestion, insomnia, anxiety, *and* tension.

BONES, JOINTS, AND MUSCLES

The health of our musculo-skeletal system is affected by how we use it: the exercise we take, our posture, and how we abuse it through over-working certain muscles and joints and neglecting others. It is also affected by our diet (see pp.26-9) and digestion. Stress and the inability to relax puts a great strain on the system and has much to answer for in the development of joint and muscle problems. If you suffer from arthritis, back pain, or sciatica you must not only examine your diet, posture, and exercise regime but also any emotional problems, and learn how you can release the tension caused by them.

ARTHRITIS AND GOUT

For rheumatoid and osteoarthritis and gout take, as *teas* or *tinctures*, a combination of celery seed, burdock, meadowsweet, and echinacea to clear waste products. For *constipation* add yellow dock root and licorice. Add a combination of devil's claw, licorice, and wild yam to reduce pain and swelling. If you are post-menopausal add hormone balancers black and blue cohosh. A good diet (see pp.26-9) should provide bone and cartilage with the nutrients for the repair process. Take supplements of cod liver oil, evening primrose oil, kelp, and selenium. To improve circulation to and from the joints take a combination of nettles, hawthorn, and prickly ash as teas or tinctures, and rub the joints with *oils* of either peppermint, rosemary, lavender, or marjoram. *Poultices* of comfrey or cabbage can bring relief.

BACKACHE AND SCIATICA

As an adjunct to other treatment, to relieve pains and stiffness, massage (see *liniment*) oils of either lavender, rosemary, marjoram, peppermint, or cloves into the area. You can also try frequent hot *compresses* of either cramp bark, valerian, chamomile, or ginger. Equal parts of *tincture* of cayenne and glycerine can also be rubbed into the area. For spinal nerve pain and sciatica rub St John's wort oil frequently into the affected part. Internally, take, as *teas* or tinctures, a combination of echinacea, couch grass, passionflower, and St John's wort. For bad pain add valerian and cramp bark.

THE AILMENTS

Quantities: See pages 15-19

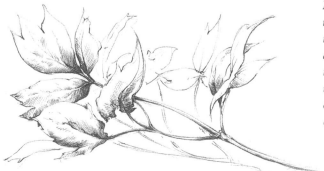

Blue cohosh (Caulophyllum thalictroides) *The root and rhizome are used, and* **actions** *are: uterine tonic, emmenagogue, anti-inflammatory, antirheumatic, antispasmodic, easing cramping in the uterus and digestive system.* **Warning** *Do not use during pregnancy, except in the last few weeks, or if you have* high blood pressure *and heart disease.*

SKIN AND EYES

The skin is our first line of defence against damage from infection, pollution, extremes of temperature and light, and physical injury, while mucous membranes protect the eyes. The skin is also a major organ of excretion and, with the kidneys, helps to regulate the water and chemical composition of the body. There is a deep connection between our nervous system and the skin, so that skin problems not only develop through physical imbalances but also from emotional problems. The skin and eyes are also affected by the circulatory and digestive systems and bowels. If these do not work properly, a system overloaded with toxins may need to excrete them via the skin.

ECZEMA

The causes of eczema are complex and need careful investigation to ensure proper treatment. An allergic reaction to substances is often involved, such as animal dander, house dust mites, wool or nylon, or to foods such as milk products, eggs, or wheat, which may need to be excluded for a few weeks. Behind this malfunction of the immune system often lie nutritional deficiencies (see pp.26-9), so take plenty of essential fatty acids in unrefined cold-pressed vegetable oils, nuts and seeds, oily fish, beans and pulses, and supplements of cod liver oil and evening primrose oil. Vitamins A, B, C, and E, and minerals zinc, magnesium, calcium, and iron are also essential (see pp.26-9). *Stress* puts further strain on the immune system and uses nutrients needed by the skin. Relaxation exercises and meditation are helpful and herbs such as chamomile, vervain, skullcap, and wild oats are calming and supportive. Take, either as hot herbal *teas* or *tinctures*, echinacea, yarrow, and chamomile for the immune system, and borage and licorice to support the adrenal glands - particularly useful when gradually reducing steroid creams. Add burdock, red clover, fumitory, and nettles to cleanse and nourish the system. Externally almond or olive oil with a few drops of chamomile or lemon balm *oil* will moisturize and soothe a dry, irritated skin. You can also use evening primrose oil, aloe vera gel, and comfrey *ointment*. If the skin is weeping or infected, add sea salt, cider vinegar, or strong pot marigold tea to a *herbal bath*, or use *compresses* of pot marigold, burdock, or yellow dock. A few drops of chamomile oil in aqueous *cream* is often very effective.

*Aloe vera The juice is used for its cathartic and emmenagogue **actions**, and the gel is emollient, vulnerary, is used to encourage skin regeneration, and is a wonderful first aid remedy. **Warning** The juice should be avoided for internal use during pregnancy and breast-feeding.*

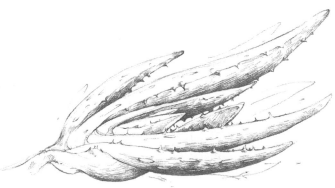

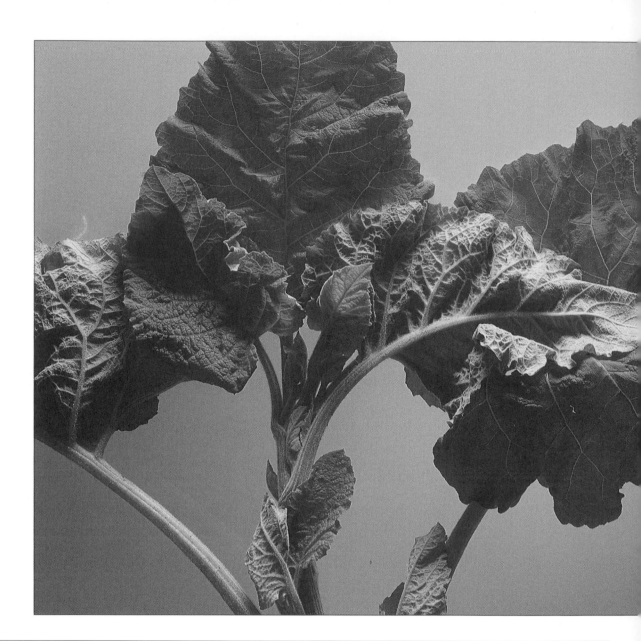

Burdock (Arctium lappa) *The roots, leaves, and seeds are all used, and **actions** are: bitter tonic, digestive, diuretic, cleansing, for skin and inflammatory joint conditions, diaphoretic, laxative, and antimicrobial. Burdock is predominantly alterative, purifying and cleansing the tissues and blood through its diuretic, diaphoretic, digestive, laxative, and antimicrobial actions. The seeds are good for treating skin* conditions such as eczema, psoriasis, boils, abscesses, and acne, *eruptions of chicken pox and measles, as well as acute infections such as* tonsillitis, colds, and flu. *The whole plant is useful during convalescence. The roots and leaves are used to treat* arthritis, rheumatism, *and* gout.

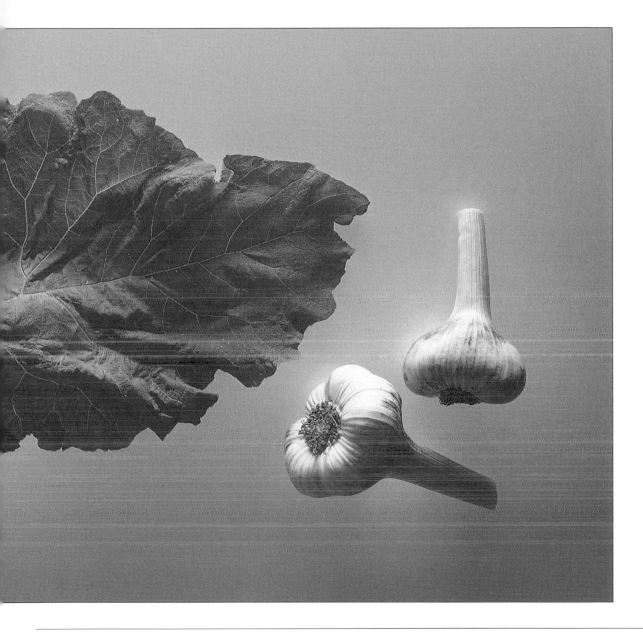

67

Garlic (Allium sativum) *The bulb is the part used, and* **actions** *are: antiseptic, antimicrobial, hypotensive, circulatory stimulant, digestive, diaphoretic, cholagogue, antispasmodic, and anthelmintic. Garlic is a most effective antimicrobial remedy, acting on viruses, bacteria, fungi, and parasites. It is used to prevent and treat* colds, flu, catarrh *and* coughs, ear *and* chest infections, diarrhoea *and* dysentery, *and* urinary tract infections, candidiasis *and* worms. *Garlic can reduce blood pressure, cholesterol levels, and tendency to clotting, making it excellent for cardiovascular disease,* high blood pressure, heart attacks, *and* strokes.

ABSCESSES, BOILS, CARBUNCLES

Never squeeze eruptions, but allow boils to come to a head and discharge on their own. You can encourage this by applying hot *poultices* for an hour or so, 3 times daily, using either marshmallow, comfrey, slippery elm, or burdock. Moisten the dried herbs and mash them in hot water (or mash and heat fresh herbs) and add a few drops of lavender, thyme, or eucalyptus *oil*, place on gauze and apply. Alternatively use equal parts of honey and cod liver oil. Continue daily until the boil has discharged and healed. Internally take *garlic* and echinacea to help resolve the infection. Take a mixture of burdock, agrimony, nettles, and poke root as hot *teas* to resolve heat and toxic congestion. If you are constipated take yellow dock root or licorice. Repeated attacks of boils indicate a run-down condition that requires further investigation and could be a sign of diabetes. **Warning** Contact your doctor if boils do not come to a head within a few days, if they develop red streaks, or if you develop a *fever*.

IMPETIGO

This infectious bacterial condition commonly affects the area around the lips, nose, and ears. Bathe the infected area with warm *teas* of either golden seal, echinacea, or pot marigold, and pat gently dry. You can also use dilute *tinctures* of pot marigold, St John's wort, or myrrh. Add a few drops of either lavender, tea tree, thyme, or eucalyptus *oil* to a bowl of hot water (to use as a steamer) or a *facial steamer*. Drink teas of a mixture of echinacea, poke root, peppermint, and burdock 3 times daily. Take *garlic* and vitamin C supplements (see p.28). Do not touch the weeping blisters as this will spread the infection, and keep your towel separate.

WARTS AND VERRUCAE

Warts are small growths composed of dead cells and caused by a virus; when they occur on the soles of the feet they are usually called verrucae. They are contagious, especially where there is moisture, for example in bathrooms and around swimming pools, so use a special plastic sock in public places and always dry the feet well. There is a variety of remedies you can apply directly to the wart – either lemon juice, garlic, the yellow juice from fresh greater celandine, the white juice from dandelion stalks, tea tree *oil*, or *tincture* of thuja. Continue daily until the wart disappears. Internally take, either as *teas* or tinctures, a combination of burdock, dandelion root, echinacea, and red clover, flavoured with licorice to enhance resistance and cleanse the system. Take regular supplements of *garlic* and vitamin C (see p.28).

Quantities: See pages 15-19

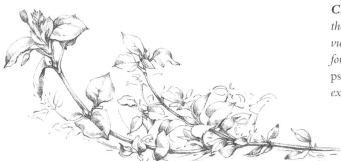

Chickweed (Stellaria media) *The aerial parts of the herb are used and the* **actions** *(externally) are: vulnerary, soothing, healing and anti-inflammatory for irritating skin conditions such as eczema and psoriasis. Internally actions are antirheumatic, expectorant, and demulcent.*

RINGWORM/ATHLETE'S FOOT

This fungal infection commonly affects the scalp, groin, and the feet, but can affect any area of the skin, hair, or nails. It is highly contagious, especially in warm, moist conditions such as around swimming pools and in bathrooms, and can be resilient to treatment. To prevent spread of infection use separate towels and wash hands after touching infected areas. Check your pets for infection as they too may need treating. Drink a mixture of echinacea, nettles, dandelion root, burdock, and peppermint *tea* to boost immunity. Externally seal the infected area off from air, to inhibit the infection, by painting on either neat lemon juice or egg white to form a glaze. Do this several times daily. Alternatively, apply neat *oils* of either lemon, lavender, tea tree, or thyme, or *tinctures* of either myrrh, echinacea, golden seal, or pot marigold 3 times daily. You can also try rubbing a garlic clove on the area. Always make sure you dry the area well, especially between the toes.

SCABIES

Caused by tiny mites burrowing into the skin, scabies is an intensely itchy condition and highly contagious. When the eggs hatch they can be passed on easily by direct contact or from bed linen, clothing (where they can survive for about 2 weeks), or from pets.

Do not scratch, as this may cause secondary infection. Take a long, hot bath at night and dry yourself briskly to open up the pores and burrows. Then apply dilute *oils* of either tea tree, bergamot, lavender, rosemary, or peppermint, or *teas* or dilute *tinctures* of either golden seal, echinacea, or poke root all over the body. Put on clean nightwear and use clean bed linen. Repeat two more nights. Internally take, as *teas* or tinctures, a combination of echinacea, cleavers, peppermint, and *garlic* perles 3 times daily. Wash all clothing, towels, and bed linen thoroughly on a hot wash, and iron them when dry, then leave 3 weeks before reusing them.

PSORIASIS

Psoriasis is a complex auto-immune skin problem that has at its origin a disturbance of the immune system, often resulting initially from *stress* or shock. Food *allergies* and nutritional deficiencies (see pp.26-9) can also play a part. Take, as *teas* or *tinctures*, herbs to relax and support the nervous system: either skullcap, vervain, wild oats, or chamomile. Combine these with either borage, wild yam, or licorice to support the adrenal glands – add a combination of burdock, poke root, red clover, nettles, and echinacea to boost immunity and cleanse the system. Support the heart and circulation, which have extra work when the skin

Vitex (Vitex agnus castus) *The folk use of this herb, also known as chaste tree, strongly suggests a hormonal effect. The fruit is used, and* **actions** *are: hormone balancer (increasing the production of luteinizing hormone and prolactin and regulating oestrogen and progesterone production), and galactagogue.*

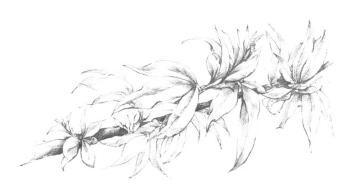

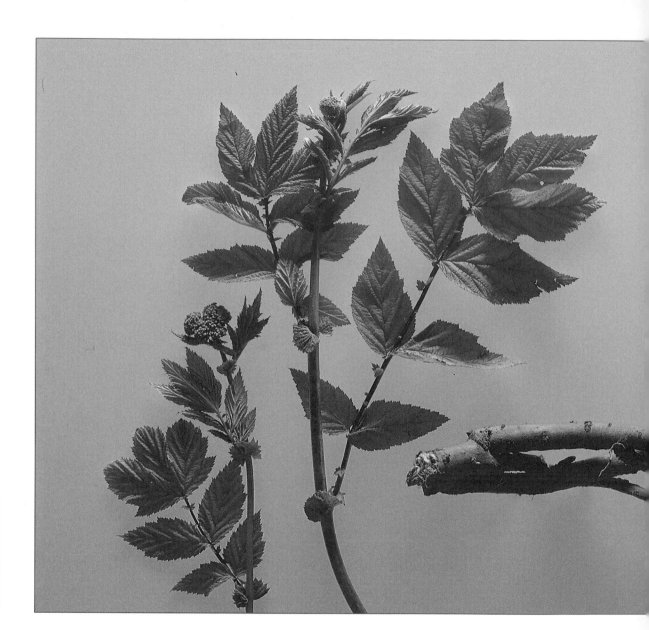

70

Meadowsweet (Filipendula ulmaria) *The aerial parts of the flowering plant are used, and **actions** are: astringent, antacid, astomachic, anti-emetic, antirheumatic, anti-inflammatory, antiseptic, diuretic, and diaphoretic. Meadowsweet has an effective anti-inflammatory action, which makes it a valuable remedy for* arthritis *and* rheumatism*. This, combined with its astringent and soothing properties, makes it* ideal for treating digestive disorders, including hyper-activity, nausea, heartburn, indigestion, gastritis, and peptic ulcers. Meadowsweet is a good remedy for diarrhoea and for reducing fevers, when given in hot infusion. It is possibly an antiseptic diuretic, useful in cystitis, and for eliminating excess uric acid associated with gout.*

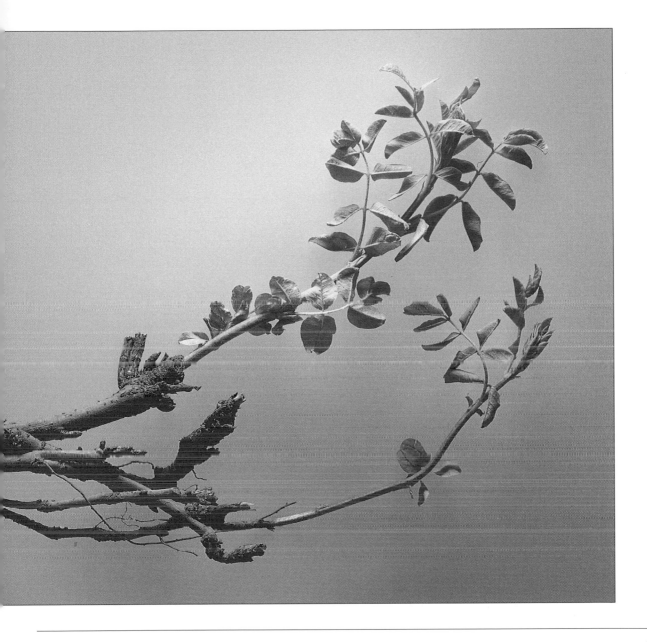

Licorice (Glycyrrhiza glabra) *The roots are used and the* **actions** *are: expectorant, febrifuge, antibacterial, anti-inflammatory, anti-allergic, oestrogenic, demulcent, antispasmodic, laxative, anti-allergic, antacid, lowers blood cholesterol, heals peptic ulcers. It can support the adrenal glands during stress and in* eczema, asthma, hay fever, arthritis, gastritis, *and* peptic ulcers. *Its soothing action in the digestive system is useful in relieving abdominal* colic, *hyperacidity,* heartburn, indigestion, *and* constipation. *While its soothing expectorant action helps* mucus/catarrh, coughs, *and* bronchitis, *its antiseptic and antibacterial actions make it an effective remedy for respiratory infections.* **Warning** *Avoid using if you have* high blood pressure, *kidney disease, or if you are pregnant.*

peels off rapidly, by adding hawthorn and motherwort. Externally comfrey *ointment*, poke root *cream*, marshmallow or chickweed ointment help to moisturize and calm the skin. Almond or olive oil, with a few drops of lavender, juniper, or bergamot *oil* can also be helpful. Add strong *infusions* of either pot marigold, yarrow, or St John's wort, or sea salt to a *herbal bath*. Sunlight can also be beneficial in clearing the skin rapidly. Take regular supplements (see pp.26-9) of kelp, vitamin C, B12, zinc, and folic acid, as well as lecithin.

CONJUNCTIVITIS AND BLEPHARITIS

In conjunctivitis the mucous membrane covering the eye becomes irritated as a result of infection, *allergy* such as *hay fever* and *rhinitis*, or pollution in the atmosphere. In blepharitis the eyelids become red and inflamed, often indicating a toxic system or allergy. For either problem bathe the eyes several times a day with eyebright *tea* - the best remedy for many eye problems. Combine it with either elderflower, chamomile, or pot marigold if you like. Always use a sterilized *eyebath* and don't use the same solution for both eyes. You can also use ordinary tea to bathe the eyes, or lie down with a warm chamomile tea bag over each eye for 10-15 minutes. Internally, take a combination of eyebright, echinacea, cleavers, burdock, and licorice as teas or *tinctures* to boost the immunity and detoxify the system. Add chamomile, golden seal, and yarrow if you have an *allergy*. Chronic conjunctivitis and blepharitis often respond well to omitting dairy products, tea, and coffee from the diet and taking supplements of cod liver oil, evening primrose oil, and vitamins C and B (see pp.26-9). **Warning** All teas used to bathe the eyes should be prepared as *decoctions* and simmered for 10 minutes to make sure they are sterilized.

EYE STRAIN OR TIRED EYES

Tired, strained eyes can be due to *stress*, debility, working long hours, particularly in air-conditioned or smoky atmospheres, under fluorescent lights, or at a computer. Try to rest your eyes at frequent intervals through the day, by closing them and covering them with the palms of your hands, and also gazing into the distance to give them a rest from close work - for several minutes at a time. Bathe the eyes with warm *decoctions* of either eyebright, pot marigold, chamomile, raspberry leaves, mullein, or elderflower several times daily, using a different solution for each eye and a sterilized eye bath. Take, as *teas* or *tinctures*, a combination of rosemary, eyebright, wood betony, vervain, and peppermint to increase the

Quantities: See pages 15-19

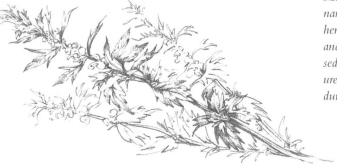

Motherwort (Leonurus cardiaca) *The common name indicates an important traditional use of the herb after childbirth. The aerial parts are used, and the **actions** are: antispasmodic, emmenagogue, sedative, cardiac tonic, short-term hypotensive, diuretic, and parturient.* **Warning** *Avoid taking during pregnancy, except to ease* childbirth.

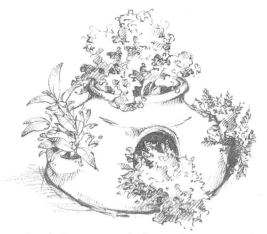

circulation to and from the eye and eat plenty of foods containing vitamins A, B, and C (see pp.26-9). It is worth getting your eyes checked by your doctor or optician if you suffer from chronic eye strain.

STYES

Styes are inflammations or infections of the glands at the base of the eyelashes that tend to occur when you are run down or tired. They are contagious, so keep your towel and washcloth separate from other people's and wash them daily, on a hot wash. Apply warm *compresses* of eyebright, burdock, or pot marigold *tea* frequently through the day. Take *garlic*, and a mixture of echinacea, burdock, golden seal, cleavers, and peppermint as teas or *tinctures*. Supplements of cod liver oil and vitamin C (see pp.26-9) will also help throw off the infection.

ACNE

Acne tends to be related to hormonal changes during adolescence and intolerance of certain foods. Avoid fatty foods and dairy produce, as well as chocolate, alcohol, sweets, red meats, iodine-rich foods, tea and coffee, and eat plenty of fresh fruit and vegetables, especially carrots. Take supplements (see pp.26-9) of zinc, cod liver oil, vitamin C, evening primrose oil and B-complex. Take, as *teas* or *tinctures*, a combination of dandelion root, burdock, nettles, cleavers, and echinacea and add yellow dock root and licorice if you are constipated. To help regulate hormonal imbalance take either vitex, wild yam, or devil's bit/false unicorn root. Try to leave your face alone and never squeeze pimples. Steam your face for 5-10 minutes once a day to clean the pores with hot *infusions* of either lavender, chamomile, yarrow, thyme, or elderflower. Wipe dry with cotton balls/wool and apply either rosewater, elderflower, distilled witch hazel, or pot marigold tea to tone and close the pores. Never use soap on your face, but if you want to wash it, use fine oatmeal mixed with water. You may need to continue treatment over several months. Once the pimples have stopped erupting use a few drops of either neroli or lavender *oil* in aqueous *cream*, or comfrey or vitamin E cream to heal the scars.

SKIN AND EYES

Eyebright (Euphrasia officinalis) *is, as its name suggests, a specific remedy for eye problems. The aerial parts of the plant are used, and the* **actions** *are: astringent, antimucous/catarrhal, and anti-inflammatory (recommended for inflammatory eye conditions),* hay fever, *and* mucus/catarrh.

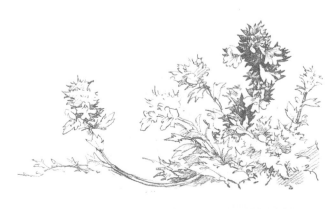

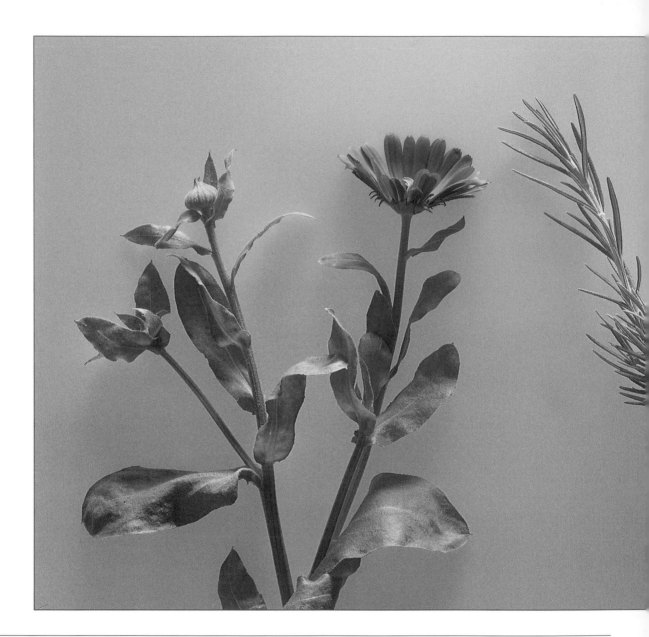

Pot marigold *(Calendula officinalis) The petals are used in herbalism, and* **actions** *are: anti-inflammatory, astringent, antiseptic, antifungal, cholagogue, emmenagogue, and vulnerary. Pot marigold is a good first aid remedy for cuts and* wounds, scalds *and* burns, bruises, insect stings, *and* bites. *It is ideal for skin problems where there is infection or injury, and can also be used for* eczema, varicose veins, varicose ulcers, *and* chilblains. *Pot marigold is valuable for* gastritis, gastric and duodenal ulcers, *and* colitis. *Its cholagogue properties are useful for* indigestion, constipation *and gallbladder problems. Its antifungal activity is useful for* thrush, *and its emmenagogue action can help* painful periods *and delayed* menstruation. **Warning** *Avoid during pregnancy.*

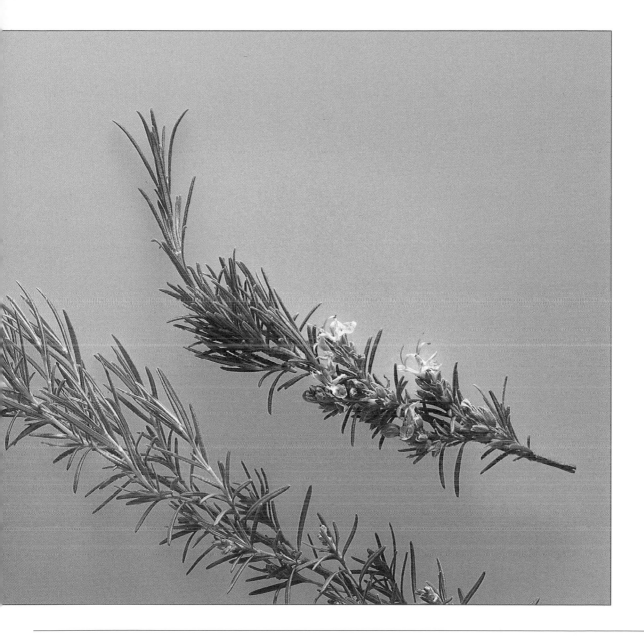

Rosemary (Rosemarinus officinalis) *The leaves are used, and the* **actions** *are: circulatory and nervous stimulant, cholagogue, carminative, antispasmodic, antidepressant, relaxant, antibacterial, antifungal, antiseptic, rubefacient, and parasiticide. Rosemary makes an excellent remedy for* headaches *and* migraine. *It acts as a circulatory and nervous stimulant, and increases the flow of digestive juices and bile. It is* useful for flatulence, indigestion, *abdominal pain or* colic, *as well as* debility, exhaustion, *poor memory and concentration,* depression *and* anxiety, *and painful periods. It relieves* poor circulation *problems such as* chilblains *and helps strengthen blood vessel walls. Externally (as an oil or liniment) it eases muscular pain,* neuralgia, *and arthritic pain.*

THE REPRODUCTIVE SYSTEM

Many imbalances of the male and female reproductive system are related to hormone imbalance. There are several herbs, notably ginseng, wild yam, blue cohosh, devil's bit/false unicorn root, and vitex that contain steroidal saponins closely resembling the human sex hormones, and have the ability to regulate hormonal activity. Stress is a major factor upsetting hormone balance, the effects of which can be minimized by the use of herbs and relaxation techniques. **Warning** Devil's bit/false unicorn root should only be used when prescribed by a herbalist.

PMS/PREMENSTRUAL TENSION

The physical, mental, and emotional changes that can occur prior to menstruation are caused by an excess of oestrogen in relation to progesterone. *Stress* and too much caffeine can also play a part, as can an overburdened liver and the use of hormones in the food industry. To balance hormones take ½tsp of vitex half an hour before breakfast, and raspberry leaves and devil's bit/false unicorn root 3 times daily as *teas* or *tinctures*. Add rosemary and dandelion root to aid liver function, and passionflower, valerian, or skullcap to ease *tension*. For *water retention* take teas or tinctures of horsetail and celery seed and reduce your salt intake. To ease *headaches* take vervain, chamomile, and rosemary. Take 2000mg of evening primrose oil in the second half of your cycle, with supplements of (see pp.26-9) calcium, magnesium, and vitamin E, and take B-complex for the whole month.

PAINFUL PERIODS

If you have intense cramps with scanty bleeding, take, as *teas* or *tinctures*, singly or in combination, prickly ash, devil's bit/false unicorn root, cramp bark, black haw, and blue cohosh with licorice 3 times daily. Add motherwort, chamomile, and skullcap if you feel very tense. Rub *oils* of chamomile, lavender, or rosemary gently into the abdomen. If pain subsides once the period starts and there is dark red blood or clots take, as teas or tinctures, wild yam, cramp bark, raspberry leaves, blackcurrant leaves, and black cohosh.

HEAVY PERIODS

Excessive bleeding from pelvic congestion can be helped by regular exercise, and a combination of brown beth/beth root, blue cohosh, agrimony, golden seal, and raspberry leaves taken either as *teas* or *tinctures*, 3-6 times daily. Capillary fragility can also be

Quantities: See pages 15-19

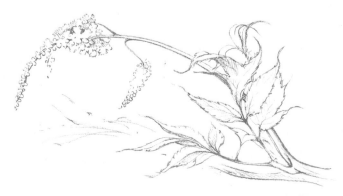

Black cohosh (Cimicifuga racemosa) *The dried root and rhizome are used, and the* ***actions*** *are: sedative, antispasmodic, anti-inflammatory, antirheumatic, hypotensive, emmenagogue, and ability to regulate uterine contractions during* childbirth. ***Warning*** *Do not use during pregnancy, except in the later stages, under the supervision of a qualified practitioner.*

responsible, so take supplements (see p.28) of vitamin C and bioflavonoids, and a combination of buckwheat tea, yarrow, limeflower, golden seal, raspberry leaves, and brown beth/beth root. For an inflammatory condition (e.g. *endometriosis* or fibroids) causing heavy periods take, as teas or tinctures, a combination of thuja, agrimony, vitex, raspberry leaves, and brown beth/beth root. For other symptoms of hormonal imbalance such as *premenstrual tension* with heavy bleeding take ½tsp vitex half an hour before breakfast, and a combination of devil's bit/false unicorn root, brown beth/beth root, squaw vine, raspberry leaves, and agrimony. You may well be anaemic, so eat plenty of iron- and vitamin-C-containing foods (see p.28) and add nettles to remedies and soups. **Warning** For constant heavy periods see your doctor.

VAGINAL INFECTIONS
To raise resistance and balance hormones take *garlic* and a combination of devil's bit/false unicorn root, echinacea, golden seal, thyme, and cleavers as *teas* or *tinctures*. Locally insert natural live yogurt, or douche with 2tsp of vinegar or lemon juice in a bowl of water twice daily. Or you can use teas or tinctures diluted in water of either pot marigold, golden seal, chamomile, or thyme, with a few drops of either thyme, oregano, or tea tree *oil* as a douche or soaked into sanitary pads and applied regularly. You can sit in a shallow *herbal bath* of any of these herbs to relieve irritation. You can also insert a clove of carefully peeled garlic (be careful not to nick it, it can burn you) twice daily. **Warning** Do not use douches if you are pregnant.

ENDOMETRIOSIS
Take a combination of vitex, devil's bit/false unicorn root, and blackcurrant leaves as *teas* or *tinctures* to rebalance hormones; add a combination of blue cohosh, cramp bark, brown beth/beth root, golden seal, and agrimony for pain and heavy bleeding. If *cramps* are severe add either passionflower, valerian, or skullcap, and massage (see *liniment*) the abdomen with *oils* of either lavender, rosemary, or chamomile. Take supplements of evening primrose oils (2000mg in the second half of the cycle), calcium and magnesium, B-complex, and zinc (see pp.26-9).

MENOPAUSAL PROBLEMS
You can help hot flashes/flushes, *depression*, *low sex drive*, palpitations, and drying of vaginal secretions by taking either singly or in combination hops, black cohosh, devil's bit/false unicorn root, and wild yam as *teas* or *tinctures*. Take these with licorice to sup-

Wild yam (Dioscorea villosa) *has traditionally been used for menstrual cramps and threatened miscarriage. The parts used are the root and rhizome, and the **actions** are: antispasmodic (for uterine and digestive colic, particularly that associated with gallstones), cholagogue, anti-inflammatory, diuretic, and antirheumatic. Small amounts may relieve* morning sickness.

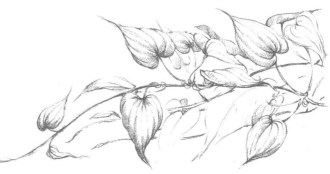

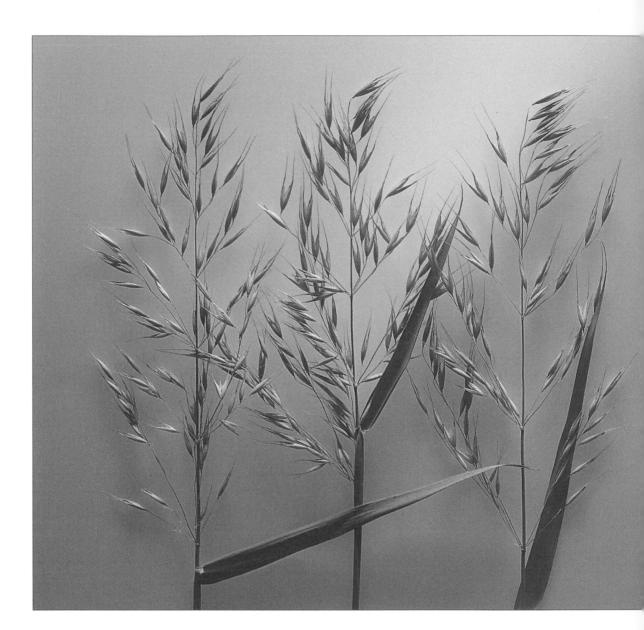

Wild oats (Avena sativa) *The seeds and the whole plant are used, and* **actions** *are: nerve tonic (specific for nervous debility, exhaustion, and convalescence), antidepressant, nutritive, demulcent, emollient, and vulnerary.   Oats are a valuable nerve tonic, and very supportive to a debilitated nervous system, during stress,* for *tension, anxiety, depression, and* exhaustion. *Their highly nutritious content makes them a good fortifying general tonic, useful when you are run down or recovering from an illness. They are also easily digested and can be used to improve digestion and treat* constipation. *The high zinc and silica content of oats gives them good healing properties: a poultice* helps relieve itchy skin and heal ulcers, as well as haemorrhoids.

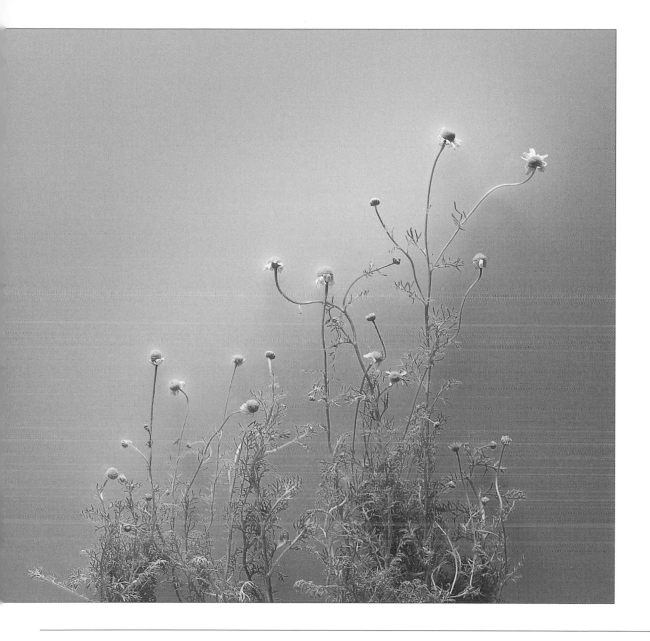

Chamomile (Matricaria chamomilla) *The flowers of the herb are used, and* **actions** *are: relaxant, sedative, analgesic, anti-inflammatory, febrifuge, antispasmodic, carminative, antiseptic, vulnerary, digestive, astringent, anti-allergic, antitoxic, antifungal, and antibiotic. Chamomile's gentle sedative and relaxant effects make it excellent for stress-related problems,* anxiety, tension, *and* insomnia, *particularly for children. It quickly reduces* fever *and induces sleep. Chamomile is one of the best remedies for* indigestion, *colitis,* diarrhoea, *and* peptic ulcers, *and it also helps relieve period pains, pre-menstrual headaches, and cystitis, and soothes conditions such as* conjunctivitis, eczema, asthma, *and* rhinitis.

port the adrenals 3 times daily. For controlling hot flashes/flushes use a mixture of sage and motherwort and up to 800 i.u. of vitamin E daily (see p.28). If you feel tired, nervous, or depressed combine St Johns' wort with other nerve tonics skullcap, wild oats, and vervain. For palpitations take hawthorn, motherwort, and lemon balm, and avoid tea and coffee. You can use comfrey *ointment*, vitamin E, and cypress *oil* for vaginal dryness.

LOW SEX DRIVE AND IMPOTENCE

For women's hormonal imbalances take a combination of devil's bit/false unicorn root, raspberry leaves, and vitex either as *teas* or *tinctures*. Add a combination of prickly ash bark, nettles, wild oats, licorice, and chinese angelica to increase vitality, and skullcap, vervain, and chamomile for *stress*. *Oils* of rose, neroli, geranium, and jasmine can be relaxing and helpful. To improve a man's libido try a combination of damiana, saw palmetto, cinnamon, licorice, and ginger. Oils of frankincense and cinnamon are beneficial. Ginseng is the remedy *par excellence* for both men and women.

LOW SPERM COUNT

Eat well (see pp.26-9), cut out junk foods and additives, alcohol, cigarettes, and caffeine and avoid tight clothes and over-hot baths. Take plenty of rest and regular exercise and supplements (see pp.26-9) of kelp, B-complex, zinc, and vitamin E. Take, either as *teas* or *tinctures*, a combination of damiana, saw palmetto, celery seeds, wild oats, licorice, and ginger 3 times daily, and *garlic* and ginseng on a regular basis. For low vitality and *stress* add a combination of nettles, skullcap, vervain, dandelion root, and prickly ash.

PROSTATE PROBLEMS

For an inflamed and infected prostate gland take couch grass, celery seed, echinacea, saw palmetto, and horsetail as *teas* or *tinctures* every 2 hours. Zinc (see p.29) is vital to male hormone balance; increase zinc intake by eating a handful of pumpkin seeds daily. Essential fatty acids are also vital - take a dessertspoon of safflower or cold-pressed linseed *oil* daily. Take plenty of exercise and take a combination of devil's bit/false unicorn root, dandelion, saw palmetto, couch grass, and prickly ash 3 times daily as teas or tinctures. **Warning** If you suspect prostate problems see your doctor.

THE AILMENTS

Quantities: See pages 15-19

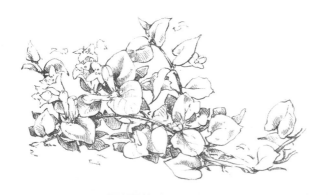

Squaw vine (Mitchella repens) *was widely used by North American Indians to prepare for* childbirth. *The leaves are used, and* **actions** *are: partus praeparator, uterine tonic, relaxant, digestive, emmenagogue, antispasmodic, diuretic, astringent, tonic, and nervous tonic.*

PREGNANCY AND CHILDBIRTH

Women all over the world have always used plants during pregnancy and childbirth to keep healthy and to prepare for the birth. Healthy eating (see pp.26-9) and taking herbs such as raspberry leaves, squaw vine, black and blue cohosh in the latter weeks of pregnancy, in conjunction with relaxation and breathing exercises can help make for a safe and easy childbirth.

MORNING SICKNESS

Chamomile, lemon balm, wild yam, raspberry leaves, and lavender, taken as *teas* or *tinctures*, all help to settle the stomach. Peppermint, ginger, cloves, cinnamon, and fennel are all warming digestives; rosemary, meadowsweet, and licorice can also help. Try sucking slippery elm tablets or sipping ginger beer (non-alcoholic). A milk- or wheat-free diet may also help.

CHILDBIRTH

For weak, ineffective contractions take raspberry leaf *tea* with a teaspoon of composition essence or a mixture of black or blue cohosh with a little ginger. A massage (see *liniment*) of dilute clove or jasmine *oil* can also help. For great *tension* and pain, and short, sharp contractions, or a rigid cervix, take blue cohosh, wild yam, cramp bark, raspberry leaves, and squaw vine either individually or combined as teas or *tinctures*. Massage the back or abdomen with dilute oils of chamomile and lavender.

BREAST-FEEDING PROBLEMS

To increase milk flow take, as *teas* or *tinctures*, either nettles, fennel, vervain, borage, raspberry leaves, or marshmallow. For sore or cracked nipples rub a drop of breast milk into the nipple after feeds, or use comfrey, pot marigold/calendula, or chickweed *ointment*, almond oil, or honey. For engorged breasts feed the baby frequently, and apply ice cold *compresses* of poke root tea, or water with a few drops of fennel, lavender, or geranium *oil*. Place fresh rhubarb or cabbage leaves inside your bra between feeds. For mastitis take a combination of yarrow, elderflower, echinacea, dandelion root, and a small amount of poke root either as teas or tinctures, and in addition, apply a warm bran or slippery elm *poultice*, or a compress of distilled witch hazel.

Brown beth/beth root (Trillium erectum) *The rhizome and root are used, and the* **actions** *are: astringent, antihaemorrhagic (particularly for profuse menstruation and post-partum haemorrhage), uterine tonic, and expectorant.* **Warning** *See your doctor immediately if you have post-partum haemorrhage.*

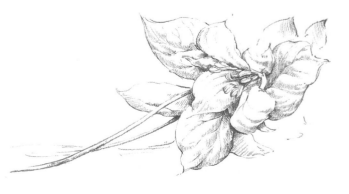

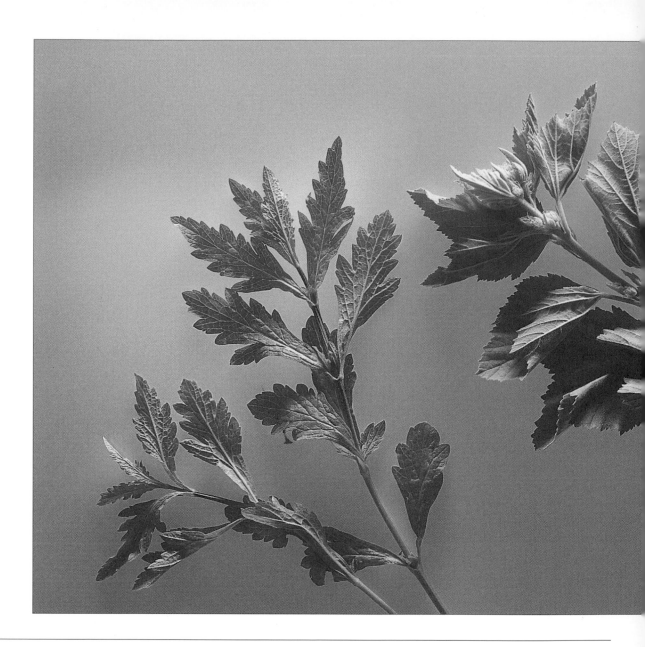

Vervain *(Verbena officinalis) The aerial parts are used and the* **actions** *are: nerve tonic, antidepressant, relaxant, cholagogue, febrifuge, diaphoretic, galacta-gogue, emmenagogue, diuretic, and antispasmodic. Vervain is an excellent tonic to the nervous system, relieving debility and exhaustion, depression, anxiety, and tension. It is helpful in liver and gallbladder disease and is beneficial in* migraines *and* headaches *of nervous and bilious origin. As a hot infusion it can reduce* fevers *and sweating, and as a* mouth-wash *it is helpful in gum disease. It increases milk flow in nursing mothers, and brings on menstruation. Its diuretic actions are helpful in* water retention *and* cystitis. *Externally it can be used for* eczema.

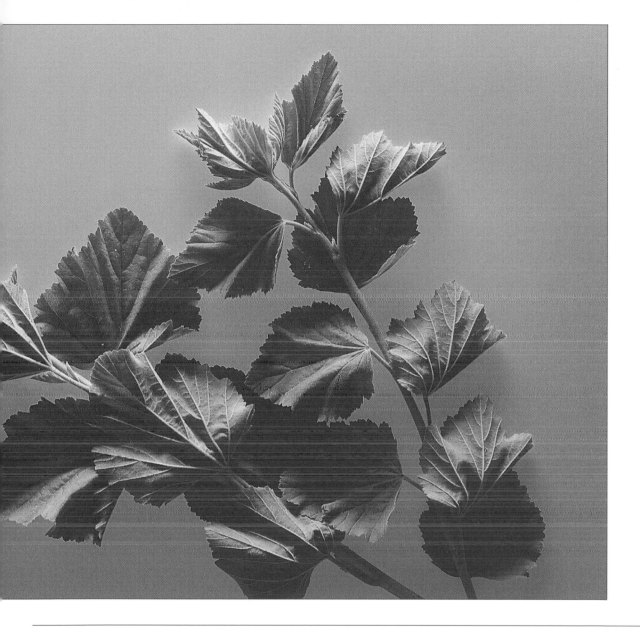

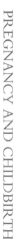

Marshmallow (Althea officinalis) *The parts used are the roots and leaves, and* **actions** *are: demulcent (soothing the respiratory, digestive, and urinary systems), diuretic, emollient, vulnerary, anti-inflammatory, and mildly expectorant. Both parts of the plant make excellent demulcent remedies, the root being used to soothe inflammatory digestive problems, such as* gastritis, peptic ulcers, colitis *and enteritis,* *and to calm skin irritation and draw out toxins from* abscesses *and* boils. *The leaf or root can be used to soothe respiratory problems such as* coughs, bronchitis, *and* catarrh, *and for inflammatory conditions of the urinary system such as* cystitis, urethritis, *and* urinary gravel. *Externally it can be used to treat* varicose veins *and* varicose ulcers.

CHILDREN'S AILMENTS

Children's ailments tend to be mild and self-limiting, and treatment is generally a matter of caring for the child, combining rest with some treatments, and basic nursing. A child's metabolism works much faster than an adult's - the breathing and heartbeat are more rapid, and a child needs proportionately more food and drink than an adult. Children become ill more rapidly, which can be worrying, but happily they also recover more quickly. In health children have far greater vital energy than most adults, which makes them very resilient in general. A wholesome diet (see pp.26-9), with plenty of essential fatty acids, proteins, vitamins and minerals, and a minimum of sugar, refined oils and junk foods, a happy family background, and healthy lifestyle will provide the basic ingredients for a robust and healthy child.

FEVERS AND INFECTIOUS DISEASES

Fever is a positive symptom of the body's fight against infection. If there is a fever over 102°F (38.9°C) bathe the child with tepid *infusions* of either yarrow, limeflower, elderflower, or chamomile to lower the temperature. You can also give these frequently as *teas* to encourage perspiration and fight the infection. Catnip, lemon balm, ground ivy, hyssop, vervain, peppermint, and meadowsweet are also beneficial, taken as teas or *tinctures*. Add echinacea to enhance immunity and give *garlic*, which encourages sweating, several times daily. Liquid is essential to encourage sweating, cool the body, and prevent dehydration, so give the child plenty to drink. Give carrot and beetroot juice to enhance the immune system, and mineral water with a little fresh lemon juice. Rest is important, so give chamomile tea to encourage relaxation and sleep. Lavender, limeflower, and lemon balm are also relaxing. You can add a few drops of essential *oil* of either lavender, chamomile, eucalyptus, or rosemary to tepid water to sponge the body, to *herbal bath* water, to *hand and foot baths*, or to liquid used to make *compresses*. Also give supplements (see pp.26-9) of cod liver oil, vitamin C, and zinc.

BEDWETTING

When this occurs regularly in a child over five who has never developed proper blad-

Quantities: See pages 15-19

Agrimony (Agrimonia eupatoria) *is an important herb with a wide range of uses, in particular it helps stop bleeding, both internally and externally, and heals ulcers. The aerial parts of the flowering plant are used and the herb's* **actions** *are: astringent, toning to mucous membranes, cholagogue, digestive and liver tonic, diuretic, and vulnerary.*

der control, there may be a physical problem that requires medical investigation. However, bedwetting can also be caused by *stress*, dietary deficiencies (see pp.26-9), particularly of calcium and magnesium, refined foods and sugar, oversensitivity to food additives, or chemicals in drinking water, or to food *allergy*. When a child starts wetting the bed after being dry, it is often due to *anxiety* or emotional problems: the child will need plenty of understanding and reassurance, perhaps even rewards for a dry bed. Avoid giving too much to drink before bed and give *teas* made from a combination of St John's wort, horsetail, and corn silk through the day and a little just before bed, sweetened with honey, to soothe an irritated or inflamed bladder. Add either skullcap, wild oats, chamomile, or lemon balm to relax and soothe the nerves. Massage (see *liniment*) *oil* of chamomile or St John's wort into the lower spine and abdomen.

HYPERACTIVITY

Hyperactivity is frequently related to food intolerance, environmental pollution, nutritional deficiencies (see pp.26-9), emotional problems, *candidiasis*, and passive smoking. If your child is very demanding, cries easily, has a poor attention span, little apparent need of sleep, and indulges in aggressive or disruptive behaviour, give supplements (see

pp.26-9) of iron, zinc, B-vitamins, magnesium, and evening primrose oil. Avoid suspect foods such as food colourings and additives, sugar, chocolate, wheat, oranges, milk, eggs, and caffeine for a while, as well as foods your child craves, and make sure meals are regular. Give, as *teas* or *tinctures*, tonic herbs for the nervous system – wild oats, vervain, and skullcap, and combine them with borage and licorice to support the adrenal glands. If you suspect the effects of pollution, or if you live in a smoky or built-up area, add red clover, kelp, and nettles to help cleanse the system of heavy metals. Breathing and relaxation exercises, music, or relaxation tapes can be helpful, as can directed and imaginative activities.

SLEEPLESSNESS

Hyperactivity, *allergy*, nutritional deficiencies (see pp.26-9), *candidiasis*, emotional *stress*, over-tiredness, and lack of fresh air and exercise can cause poor sleep patterns. Chronic problems such as irritating rashes, *asthma*, *mucus/catarrh*, or acute *infections* or *fever* can all cause disturbed nights, too. It is important to find the origins of the sleep problems to be sure of the right treatment. A healthy diet (see pp.26-9), with no junk foods, sugar, caffeine, or additives that may disturb the brain and nervous system, is vital. Increase vitamins C and B, calcium,

---

Lemon balm (Melissa officinalis) *was said, by the great Muslim physician Avicenna, to "make the heart merry". In herbalism the leaves are used, and the* **actions** *are: antispasmodic, carminative, antidepressant, diaphoretic, hypotensive, relaxant, antihistamine, emmenagogue, antiviral, and antibacterial.*

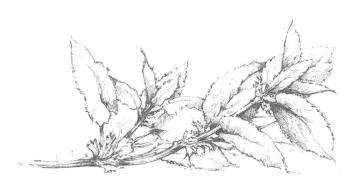

zinc, and magnesium in the diet, and avoid giving food just before bed. A warm *herbal bath* with dilute *oils* of lavender or chamomile, or strong *infusions* of either limeflower, catnip, or lemon balm will help relax the child. Massage (see *liniment*) can also be wonderfully soothing and sleep-inducing. Give a cup of warm *tea* of either catnip, lemon balm, chamomile, or cowslip flowers before bed, flavoured with licorice or honey, and give more if the child wakes in the night. You can also try a *sleep pillow* of these. If the cause seems to stem from *stress* or emotional problems, give relaxant herbs chamomile, limeflower, or skullcap through the day as well. Catnip or rosemary tea will help allay bad dreams.

CROUP

In small children a swollen larynx, blocked with *mucus/catarrh*, can impede the passage of air and cause a barking noise as the child tries to breathe. When a child wakes at night coughing, fear can often worsen the situation, so remain calm. Sit him or her up, and put a bowl or kettle of steaming water near by, or go to the bathroom and turn on the hot tap. Add to the water *oils* or strong *infusions* of either pine, eucalyptus, lavender, chamomile, or catnip, and then give chamomile *tea* to drink. You can mix oils into vaseline petroleum jelly and rub them

into the chest, or use as *compresses* to the area, or in a *vaporizer*. Over the next day or two, until the symptoms clear, give frequent teas of a mixture of catnip, chamomile, coltsfoot, marshmallow, and wild cherry, flavoured with licorice or honey. At night give the child a long, hot *herbal bath* with oils or strong infusions. Rub olive oil, with a few drops of lavender oil into the chest and give a cup of hot herb tea. Keep the air in the bedroom moist with *room sprays*.

WORMS

If you suspect your child has threadworms, check the anus carefully before bed, when the female worm migrates from the bowel to the anus to lay eggs. If your child does have worms treat any other children, and pets too. Give a cupful of balmony, peppermint, wormwood, and fennel in the morning, before eating, and repeat 2-3 times a day before meals for a week. Flavour with licorice, dilute with fruit juice, or powder the herbs in a coffee grinder and give in a teaspoonful of honey or molasses. *Garlic* is an effective remedy: give 1-2 cloves finely chopped in a spoonful of honey or a little warm milk half an hour before breakfast each day. Ground pumpkin seeds in grated carrot, which is toxic to worms, makes a good adjunct to breakfast. Check the stools daily for expelled worms and repeat the

Quantities: See pages 15-19

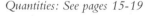

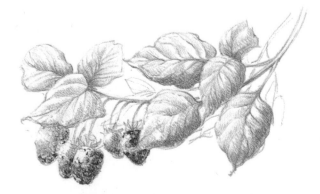

Raspberry (Rubus idaeus) *The leaves are a good astringent remedy.* **Actions** *are: astringent, uterine tonic, parturient, antispasmodic (reduces pain and eases childbirth), digestive, febrifuge, diuretic, and galactagogue.*

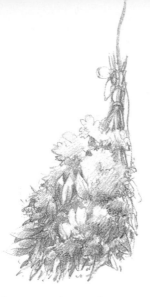

treatment after 2 weeks. Make sure children wash their hands frequently, and discourage them from scratching. Avoid sugary foods and refined carbohydrates, which worms thrive on and give live yogurt daily. Apply *oil* of either lavender, eucalyptus, thyme, or tea tree in vaseline petroleum jelly or pot marigold/calendula *ointment* to the anus at night to prevent worms from laying eggs and to relieve itching.

WHOOPING COUGH

This illness has a slow onset. It starts with a *cold* and mild *cough*. Begin treatment at the first signs of infection by giving, as *teas* or *tinctures*, elecampane, coltsfoot, and thyme, flavoured with licorice and honey, 4-6 times daily. If you mistake the first stage for a common cold and more serious coughing sets in, add to this recipe wild cherry and red clover, and if panic aggravates the spasm, add wild lettuce. You can give these every

hour if necessary. You can dilute teas with fruit juice, or use 5-10 drops of tincture in a syrup or honey. Give *hand and foot baths* of teas or dilute tinctures and use *inhalations* or *herbal baths* with strong *infusions* or tinctures in the water. You can also use essential *oils* of either thyme, cypress, eucalyptus, lavender, or marjoram as inhalations, in *vaporizers* or massage oils (see *liniment*) to the chest, abdomen, or feet. You can put a few drops on the pillow at night, or spray the room. *Compresses*, using teas, tinctures, or oils in warm water, can be applied frequently to the chest. Give *garlic* several times daily to relax the bronchial muscles and help expectoration, with supplements (see pp.26-9) of cod liver oil and vitamin C. **Warning** If you suspect your child has whooping cough, see your doctor.

DIARRHOEA

Children can easily develop diarrhoea through overeating (particularly greasy foods), fruit in season, and cold foods. It can also occur (with vomiting and *fever*) in gastro-enteritis, from taking antibiotics, from *stress* or overexcitement, or with infection. It is important to treat diarrhoea in children promptly and make sure they drink plenty to replace lost fluids. Give herbs (as listed below) every hour or two in acute diarrhoea and 3 times daily in chronic problems where

Hyssop (Hyssopus officinalis) *comes from the Hebrew name Esob and is mentioned many times in the Bible. The flowering herb is used, and the* **actions** *are: antispasmodic, expectorant, sedative, carminative, diaphoretic, antiviral, astringent, tonic, and stomachic.* **Warning** *Do not use continually for extended periods.*

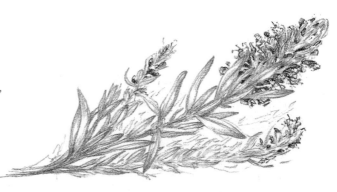

it can be related to food *allergies*, *candidiasis*, threadworms, malabsorption, or a run-down state. Give *teas* of either chamomile, thyme, peppermint, ginger, or fennel, which are mildly antiseptic and help to relieve pains. Ginger tea is especially useful when the child feels cold and looks pale, and is helpful in chronic diarrhoea associated with low vitality and digestive weakness. Chamomile and lemon balm are useful relaxants where diarrhoea is *stress*-related. Add to your chosen remedy astringent herbs: either agrimony, meadowsweet, raspberry or blackberry leaves, and soothing marshmallow. Unsweetened blackcurrant juice is useful as it contains astringent tannins and a high vitamin C content. Hot lemon and honey with a pinch of ginger or cinnamon is also a good remedy for children. Where there is *fever* give either limeflower, yarrow, or chamomile as teas or *tinctures*, and combine with antiseptic echinacea and *garlic*. Slippery elm tablets and *gruel*, as well as arrowroot, are nutritious and soothing and help the bowel retain fluid. It is best not to give solid food until the diarrhoea is better, and then give natural, live yogurt with ripe banana and brown rice, mixed with honey, before returning to normal eating. **Warning** Diarrhoea in infants is a potentially serious condition because of rapid dehydration - seek medical attention.

COLIC

Check your baby's diet, or your own if you are breast feeding, for possible irritants to the digestive tract such as cow's milk produce, wheat, or spicy foods. Give weak fennel, chamomile, hops, or lemon balm *tea* frequently. Use 1 drop of chamomile *oil* to 1pt (600ml) of warm water for a *compress* to the abdomen, which often brings quick relief. You can also massage (see *liniment*) the abdomen with dilute oils of either chamomile, lavender, lemon balm, or fennel to help relax the bowel. Catnip tea is useful for soothing a tense baby. If your baby gets colic frequently give herbal teas (1-2fl oz/28-56 ml) before each feed, and give a warm bath with strong *infusions* or oils added to the water. If you are breast feeding you can add herbs and spices to your own food to soothe the baby's gut. Ginger, carraway, dill, thyme, peppermint, fennel, and cinnamon are all useful - give as teas or *tinctures*. If you feel anxious you may be transferring *tension* to the baby; take relaxing and tonic herbs - either skullcap, vervain, wild oats, chamomile, or passionflower with licorice.

Quantities: See pages 15-19

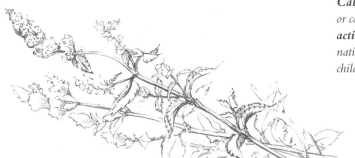

Catnip (Nepeta cataria) *is also known as catmint or catnep. The aerial parts are used, and the* **actions** *are: diaphoretic, relaxant, digestive, carminative, astringent, antispasmodic - specific for childhood infections, coughs, colds, and fevers.*

FIRST AID

People have always used remedies from the hedgerows to cure minor everyday injuries such as cuts, wounds, burns, and bites. Today this knowledge has been largely lost and most first aid remedies are purchased from the pharmacist. However, your kitchen garden, or herb and spice rack, probably contains many valuable first aid remedies that you can use simply and effectively for minor acute ailments. Put these with some basic equipment such as scissors, bandage, gauze, lint, band aids/plasters, and cotton balls/wool, and you have your first aid kit.

BRUISES

Apply a cold *compress* to contain the bruising - make this with either distilled witch hazel, 1tsp of either pot marigold or arnica *tincture* in ½pt (300ml) water, or an *infusion* of either common daisy, yarrow, or pot marigold Internally 1 drop of arnica *tincture* stirred into a glass of water will help the shock. You can also try rubbing arnica *ointment* into the bruised area.

MINOR BURNS AND SCALDS

Immerse the area in cold water for 5-10 minutes or until the pain subsides. Then apply either neat lavender *oil*, comfrey *ointment*, aloe vera juice, St John's wort oil, or pot marigold/calendula ointment. You can also use a *compress* of distilled witch hazel or an *infusion* of either comfrey, pot marigold, elderflower, or chickweed. Repeat frequently to help relieve pain, speed healing, and minimize swelling, blister formation, and prevent infection. Raise the affected part slightly to slow blood flow to the area and ease the pain. Once the pain has diminished cover loosely with a dry dressing. If the dressing sticks soak it off with a warm *decoction* of echinacea or golden seal.

MINOR CUTS AND WOUNDS

Clean the area with herbal antiseptic to prevent infection and aid healing, using 4-5 drops of either golden seal, pot marigold, St John's wort, or myrrh *tincture* in a little warm water, or an *infusion* of these herbs. If the area feels very painful bathe it regularly with diluted St John's wort tincture or *tea* of peppermint or lavender. You can also use a few drops of essential *oil* in boiled water - lavender, tea tree, peppermint, and eucalyptus are antiseptic, pain-relieving, and healing. Afterwards apply pot marigold/cal-

FIRST AID

Nettle (Urtica dioica) *grows wherever land is disturbed by humans. The aerial parts are used, and the* **actions** *(internally) are: astringent, diuretic, nutritive tonic, antirheumatic, galactogogue, hypoglycaemic, alterative, antianaemic. Externally actions are rubifacient and haemostatic.*

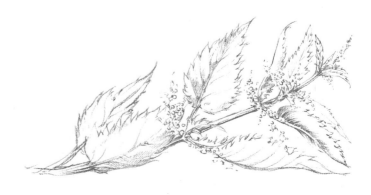

endula or comfrey *ointment*. If the cut is deep, once you have bathed it, bring the sides together and bind with surgical tape, then cover with a dressing of either honey, comfrey, or pot marigold/calendula ointment, and bandage. **Warning** Deep cuts may need to be stitched by a doctor.

SPLINTERS

Wash the area with antiseptic - a few drops of *tincture* of myrrh or pot marigold in a little water - and pull the splinter out with tweezers. If it is buried, make a warm *poultice* with either slippery elm, bread, bran, marshmallow, or comfrey root. If possible soak the area in the poultice mixture for 10-15 minutes and repeat several times through the day. Then apply comfrey *ointment* and cover with a light bandage or plaster. Once the splinter surfaces pull it out - you may need to use a needle, sterilized in a flame. Never leave a splinter untreated, as it may go septic. Should this happen crush garlic, wrap it in gauze, and bandage it on. Replace this daily and don't let the garlic contact the skin, as it may blister it. **Warning** If a splinter is large, or glass, see a doctor.

TOOTHACHE

Arrange to see your dentist, but in the meantime, to relieve the pain, try applying clove *oil* on a cotton bud to the area, or *tinc-*

ture of echinacea, both of which have anaesthetic properties. Alternatively you can use prickly ash bark - either chew it, or try it powdered, mixed with a little water, to make a paste. Take, as *teas* or tinctures, either hops, valerian, wild lettuce, or skullcap to help ease the pain.

TRAVEL SICKNESS

The best remedy for this is ginger - either chew the fresh root, or eat crystallized ginger, drink a *decoction* of ginger beer or a few drops of *tincture* in a little water. Take as frequently as you need to. Peppermint and meadowsweet *tea*, sipped often, can also help. *Inhalation* of *oils* of either aniseed, fennel, ginger, lemon balm, or peppermint will also help. If part of the problem is nerves take chamomile or skullcap.

SPRAINS AND STRAINS

To reduce pain and swelling, apply a cold *compress* of either distilled witch hazel, 1 drop of arnica *tincture* in a little water, comfrey or pot marigold *infusion*. Or make ice packs from freezing these. Then make a *poultice* of either comfrey, pot marigold, St John's wort, cabbage leaves, or daisies, and bandage the area firmly. Change the poultice twice daily. **Warning** If the pain gets worse after 24 hours consult your doctor as the underlying bone may be broken.

THE AILMENTS

Quantities: See pages 15-19

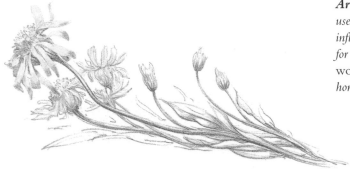

Arnica (Arnica montana) *The flower heads are used. Externally the **actions** are: vulnerary, anti-inflammatory, and antiseptic. The herb is famous for its use in homoeopathy for shock, bruises, and wounds. **Warning** Avoid internal use except in homoeopathic potency.*

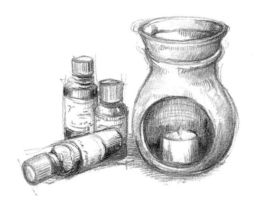

INSECT BITES AND STINGS

To relieve the pain and swelling of a bee sting, apply directly either bicarbonate of soda, sliced onion, dilute lavender *oil*, crushed garlic, or distilled witch hazel. Remove the sting by pressing it out sideways with the thumbnail, then press or suck out any poison. For wasp stings apply either cider vinegar, onion, cinnamon or lavender oil, or lemon juice. Onion, garlic, or cucumber will relieve an ant sting when rubbed into the skin. Rosemary, tea tree or lavender oil, sliced onion or garlic, or witch hazel will relieve the irritation of mosquito bites. Five drops of either citronella, tea tree, lavender, or rosemary oil in a teaspoon of base oil and rubbed on to the skin, or used in a *vaporizer*, will act as an insect repellant.

FAINTING AND SHOCK

If you feel faint sit down and put your head between your knees. Rub rosemary *oil* into the temples and inhale it from your hands. If someone has already fainted, lay them down and raise the legs. Once they have regained consciousness give sips of water or ginger *tea*, and make sure they get some fresh air. For shock take 1 drop of arnica *tincture* stirred in a glass of water and take teas of either rock rose, wild rose flower, rosemary, or elderflower. For *stress* that remains after the initial shock take, as teas or tinctures, lemon balm, chamomile, and skullcap at least 4 times daily. **Warning** This advice refers to emotional shock only, not medical shock, which can result from serious injury and requires urgent medical attention.

NOSE BLEEDS

Hold the nostrils together and lie down until the bleeding stops. Apply a cold *compress* of distilled witch hazel, yarrow, or St John's wort to the nose and the back of the neck. Alternatively, hold cotton balls/wool soaked in pot marigold *tincture* or a few drops of cypress *oil* under the nose. After the bleeding has stopped do not blow the nose or sniff as bleeding could restart. If you suffer from frequent nose bleeds take extra vitamin C and bioflavonoids (see p.28) to strengthen capillary walls. **Warning** If there is no improvement or if a nose bleed occurs after a blow to the head call your doctor.

FIRST AID

Witch hazel (Hamamelis virginiana) *is a North American Indian remedy. The parts used are the leaves and bark (also distilled witch hazel water), and the* **actions** *are: astringent- used internally for* diarrhoea *and dysentery, and externally for piles,* varicose veins, *inflammation of the eyes, throat, and skin, for* insect stings, bruises *and to stem bleeding.*

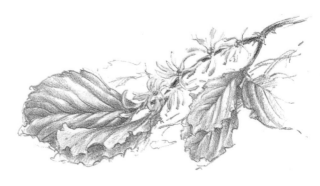

GLOSSARY/SUPPLIERS/READING LIST

GLOSSARY

Terms used to describe the actions of herbs when used as remedies:

Abortifacient Causes abortion – premature expulsion of foetus
Adaptogenic Helps to restore balance within the body
Alterative Produces gradually beneficial effects through detoxification and improving nutrition
Anaesthetic Deadens sensation and reduces pain
Analgesic Pain relieving
Anodyne Pain relieving
Antacid Reduces stomach acid
Anthelmintic Destroys or expels intestinal worms
Anti-allergic Reduces the effects of allergic reactions
Anti-anaemic Treats anaemia
Antibacterial Destroys or stops the growth of bacterial infections
Antibiotic Destroys or stops the growth of bacteria
Antimucous/catarrhal Reduces mucus/catarrh
Antidepressant Relieves symptoms of depression
Anti-emetic Relieves nausea and vomiting
Antifungal Treats fungal infections
Antihaemorrhagic Stops bleeding and haemorrhage
Antihistamine Neutralizes the effects of histamine in an allergic response
Antihydrotic Reduces or suppresses perspiration
Anti-inflammatory Reduces inflammation
Antilithic Dissolves stones or gravel in the kidneys
Antimicrobial Destroys or stops the growth of micro-organisms
Antineoplastic Has anti-cancer properties
Antirheumatic Relieves rheumatism/arthritis
Antiseptic Prevents putrefaction
Antispasmodic Prevents or relieves spasms or cramps
Antithrombotic Prevents blood clots
Antitoxic Clears toxins from the system
Antitussive Relieves coughing

Antiviral Destroys or stops the growth of viral infections
Astringent Contracts tissue, reducing secretions or discharges
Bitter Increases appetite and promotes digestion
Carminative Eases cramping pains and expels flatulence
Cell proliferator Enhances the formation of new tissue to speed the healing process
Cholagogue Increases flow of bile into the intestines
Convalescent Speeds recovery during convalescence
Demulcent Soothes irritated tissues, especially mucous membrane
Depurative Cleanses and purifies the system, especially the blood
Diaphoretic Promotes perspiration
Digestive Aids digestion
Diuretic Promotes the flow of urine
Emetic Causes vomiting
Emmenagogue Promotes menstrual flow (avoid in pregnancy)
Emollient Soothes and heals the skin
Expectorant Promotes expulsion of mucus from the respiratory tract
Febrifuge Reduces fever
Galactagogue Increases flow of milk
Haemostatic Stops bleeding and haemorrhage
Hormone balancer Improves hormone balance
Hypnotic Induces sleep
Hypoglycaemic Reduces blood sugar
Hypotensive Reduces blood pressure
Immune enhancer Helps the functioning of the immune system
Laxative Promotes evacuation of the bowels
Narcotic Relieves pain and induces sleep
Nervine Calms the nerves
Nutritive Contains nutritious substances
Oestrogenic Resembles the actions of oestrogen
Oxytocic Stimulates contraction of uterine muscle and so facilitates childbirth
Parasiticide Kills parasites
Parturient Facilitates childbirth
Partus praeparator Prepares for childbirth
Purgative Produces vigorous

emptying of the bowels
Relaxant Relaxes nerves and muscles
Restorative Restores normal physiological activity
Rubefacient A gentle local irritation that produces redness of the skin
Sedative Reduces nervousness and anxiety, induces sleep
Stimulant Produces energy
Stomachic Stimulates, strengthens, or tones the stomach
Styptic Stems bleeding
Sudorific Promotes perspiration
Tonic Invigorates and tones the body and promotes a feeling of wellbeing
Vasodilator Widens blood vessels, lowering blood pressure
Vulnerary Promotes healing of wounds

HERB SUPPLIERS AND ORGANIZATIONS

Andre Viette Farm and Nursery, Route 1, Box 16, Fishersville, VA 22939
Tel: (703) 943-2315

Aphrodisia,
282 Bleeker Street, New York, NY 10014
Tel: (800) 221-6898

The Herb Society of America, 9019 Kirtland, Chardon Rd, Mentor, Ohio 44060

ABC Herb Nursery,
PO Box 313, Lecoma, MO 65540

Brooklyn Botanic Garden, 1000 Washington Avenue, Brooklyn, New York, NY 11225

Companion Plants,
Route 6, Box 88 Athens, Ohio 45701

Earthstar Herb Gardens, 438 W Perkinsville Rd, Star Route 1, Box 82, Chino Valley, Arizona, AZ 86323

Frontier Co-operative Herbs
Box 299, Norway, IA 52318
Tel: (319) 227-7991

Nichols Garden Nursery,
1190 North Pacific Highway,
Albany,
OR 97321
Tel: (503) 928-9280

Owens Farms,
Curve Nankipoo Road,
Route 3, Box 158A,
Ripley, TN 38063
Tel: (901) 635-1588

READING LIST

Chaitow, Leon, *Clear Body, Clear Mind*, 1990, Unwin Hyman, UK; Greenhouse, Australia; and as *The Body/Mind Purification Program*, Simon & Schuster, US

Christopher, Dr J., *School of Natural Healing*, 1976, Biworld

Davis S. and Stewart A., *Nutritional Medicine*, 1987, Pan Books

De Bairacli Levy, Juliette, *The Illustrated Herbal Handbook*, 1991 Faber & Faber

Grieve, Mrs M., *A Modern Herbal*, 1990, Penguin Books

Griggs, Barbara, *Green Pharmacy*, 1981, Norman & Hobhouse

Jarmey, Chris, and Tindall, John, *Acupressure for Common Ailments*, 1991, Gaia Books UK; Simon & Schuster, US; Angus & Robertson, Australia

Kirsta, Alix, *The Book of Stress Survival*, 1986, Unwin Hyman, UK and Australia; Simon & Schuster, US and Australia

Lam, Master Kam Chuen, *The Way of Energy*, 1991, Gaia Books, UK; Simon & Schuster, US and Australia

Lidell, Lucy, *The Book of Massage*, 1984, Ebury Press, UK and Australia; Simon & Schuster, US

Lidell, Lucy, *The Sensual Body*, 1987, Unwin Hyman, UK and Australia; Simon & Schuster, US

Lust, John, *The Herb Book*, 1974, Bantam Books

Mabey, Richard (consult ed), *The Complete New Herbal*, 1988, Elm Tree Books, UK; and as *The New Age Herbalist*, Collier Books, US

McIntyre, M., *Herbal Medicine for Everyone*, 1988, Penguin

Messegue M., *Health Secrets of Plants and Herbs*, 1981, Pan Books

Mindell, Earl, *Earl Mindell's Herb Bible*, 1992, Simon & Schuster

Nagarathna, R, Nagendra, R and Monro, Robin, *Yoga for Common Ailments*, 1991, Gaia Books, UK, Simon & Schuster, US; Angus & Robertson, Australia

Palaiseue J., *Grandmother's Secrets*, 1973, Barrie & Jenkins

Price, Shirley, *Aromatherapy for Common Ailments*, 1991, Gaia Books, UK; Simon & Schuster, US; Angus & Robertson, Australia

Scheffer, M., *Bach Flower Therapy*, 1986, Thorsons

Scott, Julian. *Natural Medicine for Children*, 1990, Unwin Hyman, UK and Australia; William Morrow/Avon Books, US

Scott, Julian and Susan, *Natural Medicine for Women*, 1991, Gaia Books, UK; Avon Books, US; Simon & Schuster, Australia

Sivananda Yoga Centre, *The Book of Yoga*, 1983, Ebury Press, UK and Australia; and as *The Sivananda Companion to Yoga*, Simon & Schuster, US

Stanway, Dr Andrew (gen ed), *The Natural Family Doctor*, 1987, Century Hutchinson, UK; Simon & Schuster, US

Stanway, Dr Penny, *Diet for Common Ailments*, 1989, Sidgwick & Jackson, UK; Angus & Robertson, Australia; and as *Foods for Common Ailments*, Simon & Schuster, US

Thomas, Sara, *Massage for Common Ailments*, 1989, Sidgwick & Jackson, UK; Simon & Schuster, US; Angus & Robertson, Australia

Thomson W., *Healing Plants*, 1978, Macmillan

Weiss, F., *Herbal Medicine*, 1988, Arcanum

Worwood, V., *The Fragrant Pharmacy*, 1990, Macmillan

INDEX

Publisher's acknowledgments
Gaia would like to thank: Lucy Lidell, Lesley Gilbert, Susan Walby, Libby Hoseason, Susan Mennell, Helen Spencer, Phil Gamble, Philip Dowell, Barbara Dowell, Dr Richard Donze, David Johnson for the contents page photographs, Norfolk Lavender (suppliers of genuine English lavender oil) for permission to use the title page photograph. For plants and reference material: Dorothy Bollen, Richard Lewin of Salley Gardens, Caroline and John Stevens of Suffolk Herbs, Tricha Menist of Southwick County Herbs, and the Herbary Prickwillow, Ely.

Author's acknowledgments
The author would like to thank Sally Lyons for her interest and support and for typing the manuscript, and Graeme Garden for reading it.

BESTSELLING BOOKS FOR THE HEALTH OF BODY AND MIND
THE GAIA SERIES - FROM FIRESIDE BOOKS

FOODS FOR COMMON AILMENTS
by Dr. Penny Stanway
This concise guide gives advise on how to use everyday foods to prevent and treat 80 common health problems—from acne to migraine, and more.
0-671-68525-2, $10.95 ❏

MASSAGE FOR COMMON AILMENTS
by Sara Thomas
How to use the healing power of your hands to relieve everyday disorders—from asthma to menstrual discomfort, and more.
0-671-67552-4, $9.95 ❏

THE BODY/MIND PURIFICATION PROGRAM
by Dr. Leon Chaitow
This guide provides a holistic plan for detoxifying and re-energizing your life through various techniques such as massage, meditation, breathing exercises, special diets and more.
0-671-68526-0, $13.95 ❏

THE NATURAL HOUSE BOOK
by David Pearson
foreword by Malcolm Wells
Combining home design with health and environmental concerns, this lavishly illustrated, comprehensive handbook shows you how to turn any house or apartment into a sanctuary for enhancing your well-being.
0-671-66635-5, $18.95 ❏

THE BOOK OF MASSAGE
by Lucy Lidell
From massage to shiatsu and reflexology, this book teaches you the power of the human touch.
0-671-54139-0, $13.95 ❏

THE WAY OF ENERGY
by Master Lam Kam Chuen
The first step-by-step guide to this unique and highly praised form of ancient Chinese medicine—motionless exercises that cleanse and strengthen your body and actually generate energy.
0-671-73645-0, $14.95 ❏

AROMATHERAPY FOR COMMON AILMENTS
by Shirley Price
This first-of-its-kind guide shows how to apply thirty of the most versatile essential oils to treat more than forty common health problems.
0-671-73134-3, $11.95 ❏

THE BOOK OF STRESS SURVIVAL
by Alex Kirsta
Learn how to relax and stress-proof your lifestyle with this comprehensive reference on stress and management.
0-671-63026-1, $13.95 ❏

THE SENSUAL BODY
by Lucy Lidell
Reawaken your sensual self with this unique guide to mind-body exercises from around the world.
0-671-66034-9, $11.95 ❏

THE WAY OF HARMONY
by Howard Reid
A guide to self-knowledge and inner strength through the arts of T'ai Chi Chuan, Hsing I, Pa Kua, and Chi Kung.
0-671-66632-0, $12.95 ❏

ACUPRESSURE FOR COMMON AILMENTS
by Chris Jarmey and John Tindall
A step-by-step, instructional guide that demystifies this ancient healing art, teaching readers techniques to treat over 40 chronic and acute ailments.
0-671-73135-1, $11.95 ❏

THE NATURAL FAMILY DOCTOR
by Andrew Stanway, M.B., M.R.C.P. and Richard Grossman
An encyclopedic self-help guide to homeopathy, acupuncture, herbalism, therapeutic touch, and more.
0-671-61966-7, $12.95 ❏

YOGA FOR COMMON AILMENTS
by Dr. Robin Monro, Dr. Nagarathna and Dr. Nagendra
From cancer to the common cold—this holistic guide shows you how to use yoga to reduce inner tensions and heal the body naturally.
0-671-70528-8, $10.95 ❏

MAIL THIS COUPON TODAY - NO-RISK 14-DAY FREE TRIAL

Simon & Schuster Inc.
200 Old Tappan Road
Old Tappan, NJ 07675, Mail Order Dept.

Please send me copies of the above titles. (Indicate quantities in boxes.)
(If not completely satisfied, you may return for full refund within 14 days.)
❏ Save! Enclose full amount per copy with this coupon. Publisher pays postage and handling; or charge my credit card.
❏ Mastercard ❏ Visa
My credit card number is_____ Card expires_____
Signature_____
Name_____
Address_____
City_____ State_____ Zip Code_____
or available at your local bookstore   Prices subject to change without notice